Essentials of

DENTAL CERAMICS

An Artistic Approach

Essentials of Dental Ceramics: An Artistic Approach

GERARD J. CHICHE, D.D.S.
Associate Professor
Louisiana State University
School of Dentistry
New Orleans, Louisiana

ALAIN PINAULT
Master Dental Ceramist
Paris, France

YEAR BOOK MEDICAL PUBLISHERS, INC.
CHICAGO • LONDON • BOCA RATON

2 3 4 5 6 7 8 9 0 R K 92 91 90

Library of Congress Cataloging-in-Publication Data

Chiche, Gerard J.
Essentials of dental ceramics : an artistic approach / Gerard J. Chiche, Alain Pinault.
p. cm.
Includes bibliographies and index.
ISBN 0-8151-1666-7
1. Dental ceramics. I. Pinault, Alain. II. Title.
[DNLM: 1. Dental, Partial. 2. Dental Porcelain. 3. Dental Restoration, Permanent—methods. WU 515 C533e]
RK655.C47 1988 88-5682
617.6'75—dc19 CIP
DNLM/DLC
for Library of Congress

Sponsoring Editor: David K. Marshall
Associate Managing Editor, Manuscript Services: Deborah Thorp
Production Project Manager: Gayle Paprocki
Proofroom Supervisor: Shirley E. Taylor

To Lynn
To Monique

FOREWORD

Dr. Gerard Chiche, previously a Louisiana State University School of Dentistry graduate student from Paris, and now a faculty member at that institution since 1982, is a once-in-a-lifetime student. Dr. Chiche has developed into a fine clinician, teacher, lecturer, writer, and photographer, as this book will disclose. Writing in a second language is a major accomplishment in itself. He has achieved his goal as a result of long hours of work.

This book will be a major contribution to the dental profession, dental technology, and laboratory personnel in the development of finer dental ceramics esthetics. It is a basic manual for those needing to refine dental ceramics techniques.

Edmund E. Jeansonne, D.D.S.
Dean Emeritus
Louisiana State University
School of Dentistry
New Orleans, Louisiana

FOREWORD

With the introduction of castable glass ceramics and porcelain veneers, it is natural that attention should be concentrated on these new technologies. However, the full porcelain veneer crown will remain the basic restoration for successful esthetic dentistry, and this timely book by Gerard J. Chiche and Alain Pinault reminds us that all dentists and technicians must return to fundamental principles when constructing ceramic restorations. The book reflects the authors' expertise, and it is refreshing to see that these young ceramists are continuing the tradition of high quality ceramics that has been prominent at Louisiana State University School of Dentistry.

The beginner should gain confidence when reading this book, since the high standard of work shown in the illustrations is an example of what dedication by these two young Frenchmen can achieve in a comparatively short period. Their impact on the dental scene is assured.

John W. McLean, O.B.E., F.D.S., R.C.S. (Eng.), M.D.S., D.Sc. (London), Dr. Odont. (Lund)

Consulting Professor in Fixed Prosthodontics and Biomaterials
Louisiana State University
School of Dentistry
New Orleans, Louisiana

PREFACE

Increased esthetic demands by the public have resulted in the setting of new quality standards in dental ceramics, orientating the dental profession toward development of new and improved ceramic systems in terms of tensile strength and translucency. The ceramometal restoration remains the main standard for daily bridge work and must rely on intricate building techniques to compensate for its intrinsic esthetic limitations.

The purpose of this textbook is to cover the fundamental artistic principles governing sculpturing and building of dental porcelain in our laboratory. It is devised in a progressive format with numerous intentional repetitions and systematic overlapping from one chapter to the next. The book focuses on the "live at the bench" detailed construction of four typical clinical situations, and should also serve as a useful reference to the clinician for a better understanding of shade prescription and its translation into the ceramic buildup. Essentials of dental anatomy, occlusal waxing, casting, and framework design are all prerequisites not within the scope of this textbook.

Emphasis is placed on creation and preservation of translucency and internal development of color, whereas extrinsic staining is a useful adjunct when applied sparingly, but by no means is a panacea. All these guidelines apply to most of the commercially available dental ceramics with slight variations so that the reader may concentrate on the brand of his choice.

Gerard J. Chiche, D.D.S.
Alain Pinault

ACKNOWLEDGMENTS

Louisiana State University has always been strongly committed to teaching dental ceramics in depth, at both the undergraduate and the postgraduate levels, thanks to the unselfish dedication of Dr. Edmund E. Jeansonne, Dean Emeritus, and Dr. H. Bruggers, Associate Dean. This textbook is our contribution to their endeavors. Dr. John McLean's principles and techniques have been a fundamental source of inspiration since our introduction to dental ceramics and remain a constant reference for our work.

We would like to sincerely thank Dr. J. D. Harrison, Chairman of Fixed Prosthodontics at Louisiana State University, for his encouragement and guidance in this project, which also owes so much to the invaluable technical assistance of Larry LaHoste, C.D.T., Head of the Dental Ceramics Laboratory, Ron Elliot, and Gary Bird, C.D.T. from Unitek Corporation.

We would like to acknowledge the teachings of Dr. Jack Preston, Dr. Ronald Goldstein, Dr. Harold Shavell, Dr. Lloyd Miller, and the wonderful artistry of Willy Geller and Makoto Yamamoto.

Finally, a lot of our gratitude goes to Shawn Brandt for all her efforts in preparing and editing all the manuscripts.

Gerard J. Chiche, D.D.S.
Alain Pinault

CONTENTS

Chapter 1

Instrumentation

From an artistic standpoint, dental ceramic technology relies strictly on the quality of the instrumentation. Handling of porcelain requires discipline for optimum control and maximum speed. A specific instrument must be selected according to the size of the increment and the delicacy required for buildup. The respective size, flexibility, and density of a brush dictates a precise purpose. Always bear in mind that in most instances blades or carving points—and, after firing, rotary stones—cannot substitute for the skillful use of the brush.

The following instruments for mixing, building, and condensing are recommended.

BUILDUP AND OPAQUE BRUSHES

The Buildup Brush (Sable Hair No. 6).— This is the most versatile brush (Fig 1–1). It is large enough to retain sufficient water to apply major increments of porcelain, yet its end can be shaped into a fine tip that allows for precise and delicate additions (Fig 1–2). The length and density of the brush provide for optimum rigidity, whereas the residual flexibility facilitates its control. By using the body of the brush as a reservoir for water and shaping the end into a fine point, a penlike effect is created, always feeding water to the buildup. The finer the point, the better the regulation of water exiting the tip. Any entrapped air between the bristles should be eliminated before any porcelain is applied, by rubbing the brush against the wall of a stainless steel water bowl. Next, resharpen the tip by rotating it onto tissue paper. It is now ready for a new addition. Never use this instrument with opaque powder since residues may eventually mix with enamel and dentin powder.

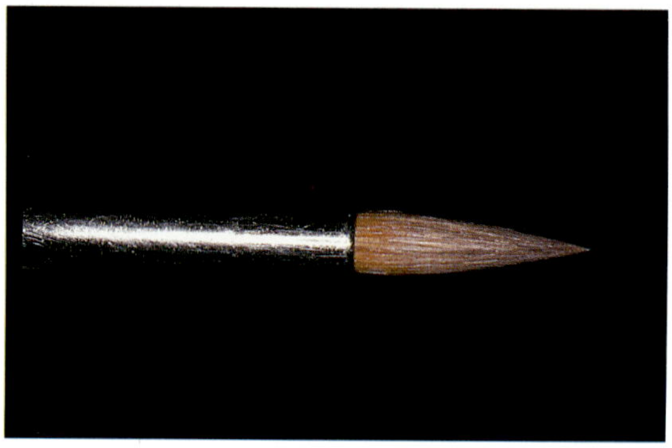

FIG 1–1

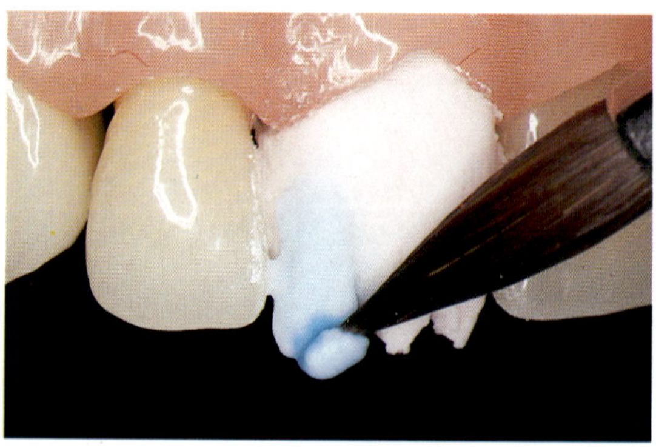

FIG 1–2

Large Soft-Hair Brush.— This brush is very soft and flexible. The polishing strokes are worked from only a cervicoincisal direction to direct, realign, or highlight the axial morphology (Fig 1–3). The strokes also cause some vibrations, which reactivate water to the surface of the buildup and facilitate the next addition. Some sculpturing action is also possible to a somewhat limited extent.

Fine Sable-Hair Brush.—This brush is very useful for fine occlusal additions (Fig 1–4) and occlusal grooving because of its high density and maximum water retention, which make it possible to readily blend a very small addition to the buildup by surface tension without dehydration. It is recommended for fine, delicate applications for which greater control is required.

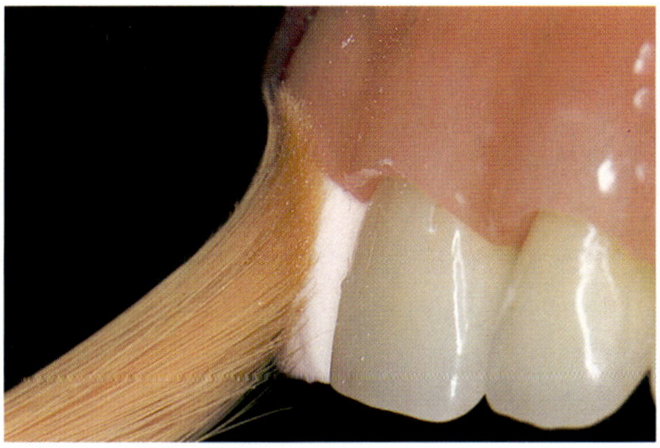

FIG 1–3

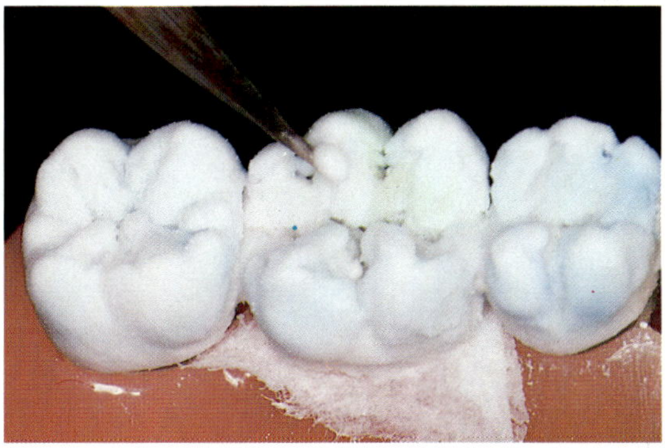

FIG 1–4

Opaque Brush.—This is reserved exclusively for opaque manipulation. Work its whole length from the base to the tip to pick up the opaque mixture in a spatula-like action (Fig 1–5). The respective sizes of the buildup brush, fine sable-hair, and opaque brush are depicted from left to right in Figure 1–6.

STAINING BRUSHES (Fig 1–7)

Fine Staining Sable Brush.— Use its whole length in a brushing stroke to emphasize a fine embrasure space with surface colorant. This brush is reserved mainly for the interproximal embrasures.

Extra Fine Staining Sable Brush.—This brush is very short and very rigid. Its very fine tip is meant to highlight the inner aspect of occlusal pits with surface colorants.

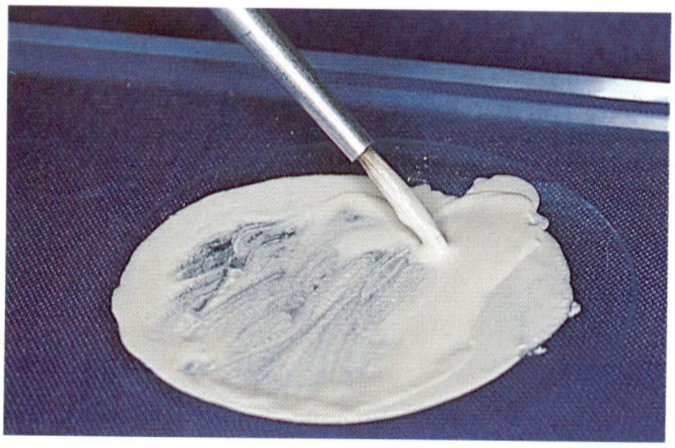

FIG 1–5

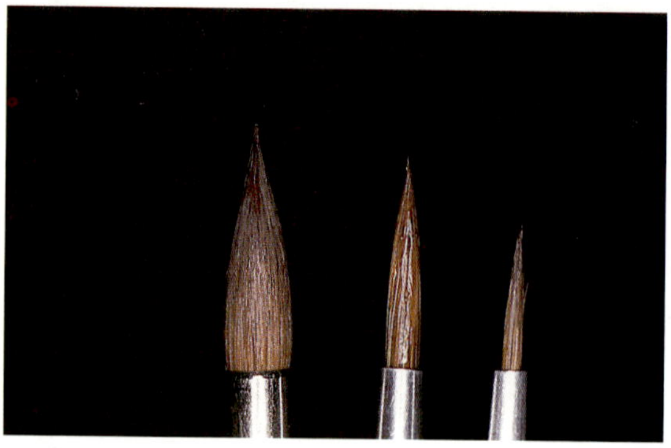

FIG 1–6

CARVING AND GROOVING BLADES (Fig 1–8)

Carving Blade.—This instrument is custom made by mounting a semirigid razor blade onto a wooden handle. The gross axial outlines are carved with overlapping sweeping strokes. All labial and incisal cutbacks are performed in the same fashion (Fig 1–9). With straight vertical motions it creates individualization between every bridge unit, especially in the anterior region.

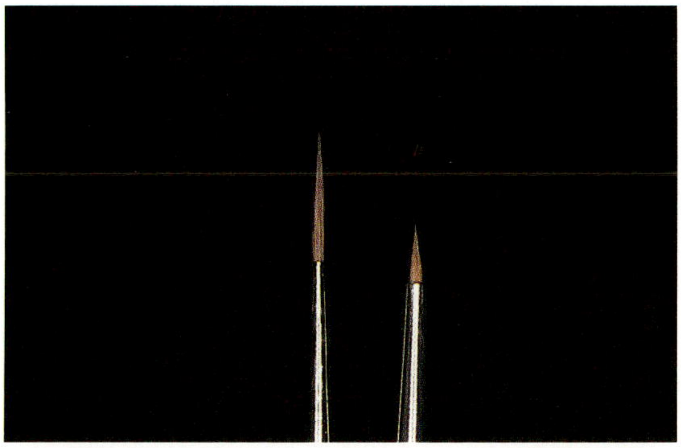

FIG 1–7

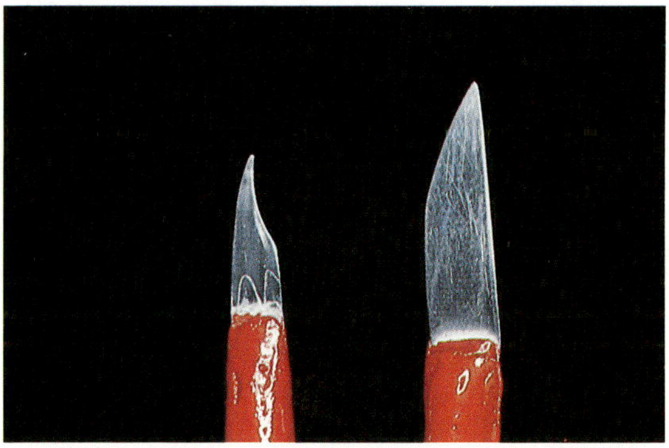

FIG 1–8

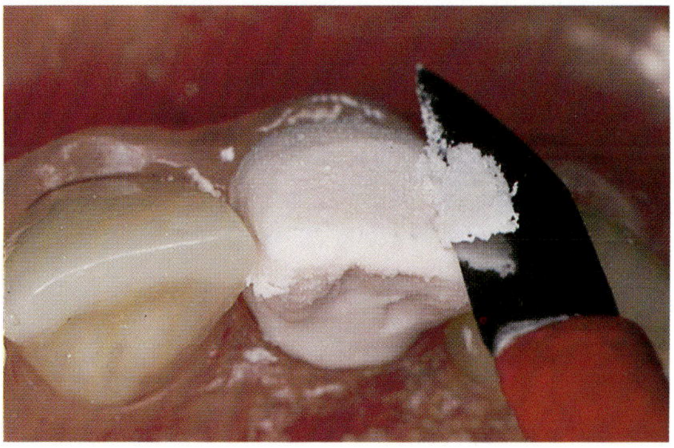

FIG 1–9

Grooving Blade.—The grooving blade is another customized razor blade over a wooden handle. It occupies very little space when carving because of its very fine tip. It deepens and emphasizes primary and accessory occlusal grooves. Its curved edge is ideal for occlusal cutback of posterior teeth (Fig 1–10) and lingual cutback of anterior teeth.

ASSORTED OTHER TOOLS

The Mixing Spatula.—This allows for both precise dispensing of the powder from the bottle to the glass plate and its mixing with liquid binder. Trenches are first created in the powder to facilitate irrigation and wetting (Fig 1–11). It is then quickly saturated with liquid with a few gentle taps of the flat end of the spatula. A satisfactory mix must be creamy and heavily saturated so that it

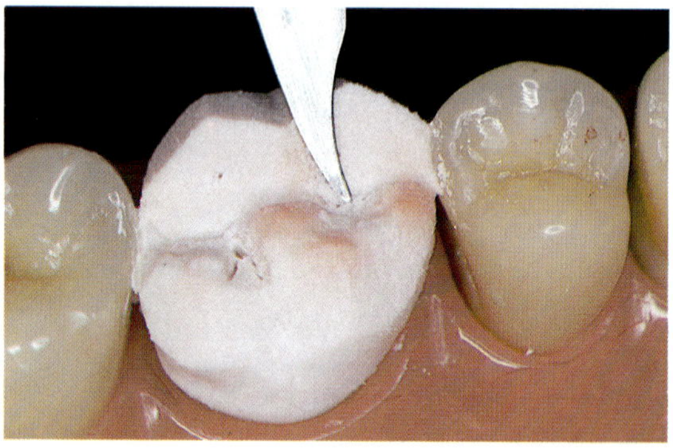

FIG 1–10

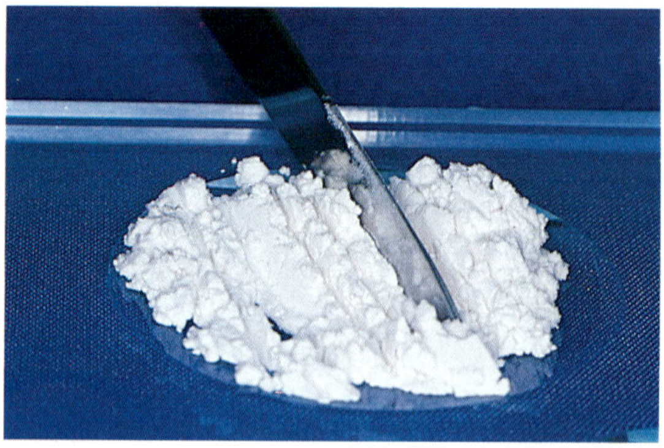

FIG 1–11

will not readily run when lifted from the glass plate (Fig 1–12). Do not overstir, since this will incorporate air bubbles. Unlike the technique for mixing dental cements, the spatula should never be allowed to scrape the glass plate since metal oxides from its surface can easily contaminate the mixture.

Insert next the buildup brush at a 45–degree angle between the glass plate and the porcelain mix. The length of its penetration controls precisely the size of the bead to be picked up (Fig 1–13).

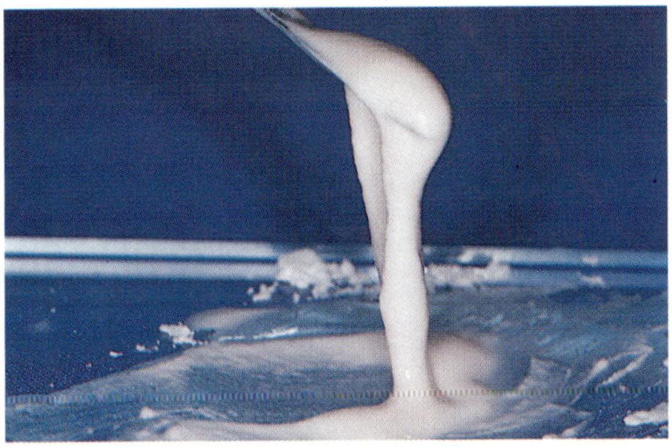

FIG 1–12

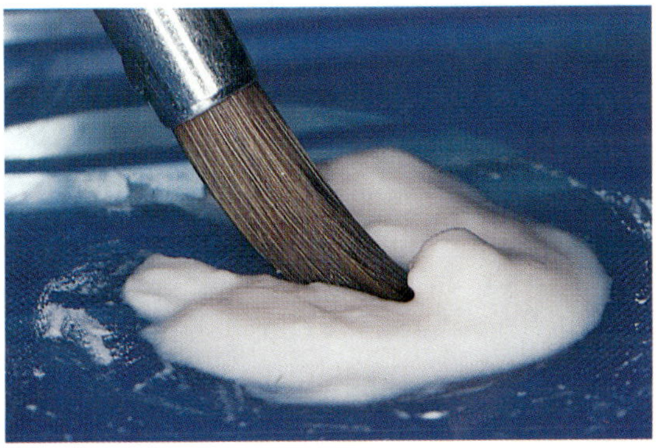

FIG 1–13

The Ceramosonic Condenser (Fig 1–14).— This provides for fine continuous vibrations of 8– to 10–μm amplitude at a frequency of 20,000 to 28,000 Hz.[1] This small amplitude promotes good packing density without displacement or intermixing of the built-in colors or distortion of the whole buildup. One- or 2–second applications are sufficient for body condensation. It is used more deliberately with opaques and porcelain margin powders.

Modified Pliers.— A regular cotton pliers is adjusted at each end with two additional bends and converted into an automatic plier that can hold a casting from its internal aspect (Fig 1–15). It is especially useful when there is little or

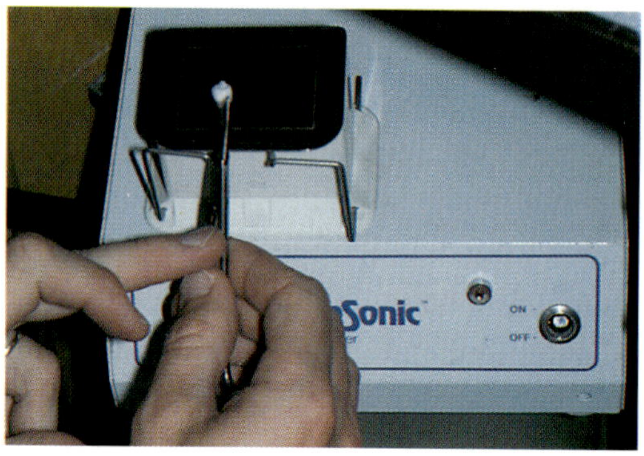

FIG 1–14

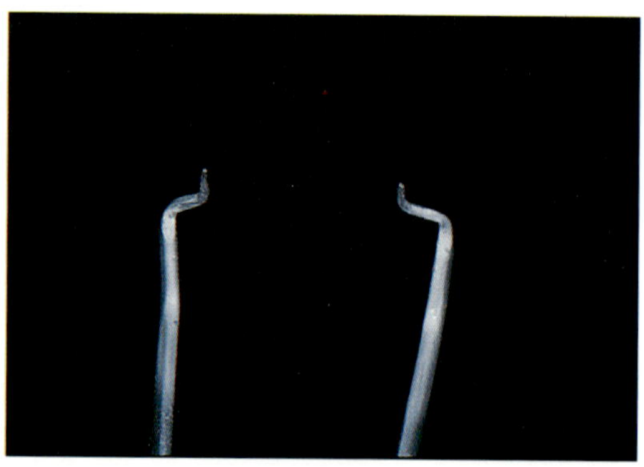

FIG 1–15

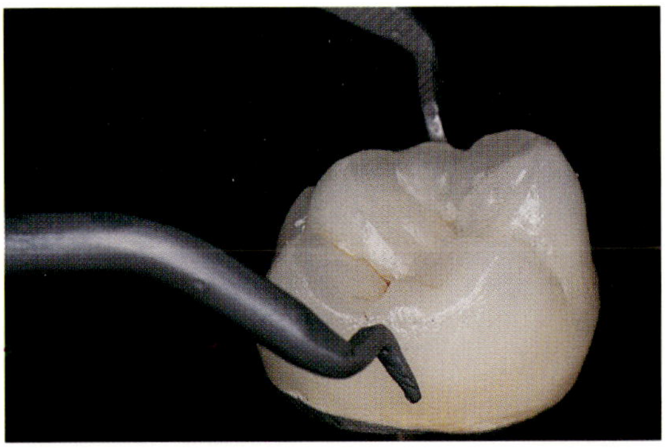

FIG 1–16

no metal collar available for prehension with a hemostatic pliers during addition and correction of interproximal contacts, for carrying the unfired crown to the firing tray, and for internal prehension after surface colorants are painted (Fig 1–16).

REFERENCE

1. Kuwata M: *Color Atlas of Ceramo-metal Technology*. St Louis, Ishiyaku Euro America, 1986, vol 2.

Chapter 2

Opaque Condensation

The purpose of the opaque coating is to mask the metal background. It is essential to fulfill this goal with the thinnest possible layer for the following three reasons:

1. Adequate shade reproduction depends on the remaining thickness of dentin and enamel. This is critical with lighter shades, which require more thickness than darker ones.[1]
2. Opaque reflectivity is detrimental and unavoidable. It can be compensated for by promoting subsurface refraction and light scattering through the dentin and enamel layers, provided they are of sufficient thickness.
3. Thicker opaque is brighter. Manufactured opaques with the best masking ability also tend to be brighter, whereas opaques with lesser masking ability have a lower value. The latter type is preferred when compensations for brightness in the body porcelain are desirable, especially in the cervical area where thickness is limited.

Two separate opaque coatings and firings are necessary. Thickness and uniformity are better controlled and more easily achieved.[2] A single application would prove very difficult without stagnation, localized thickening, and air entrapment, which could resurface at a subsequent firing.

FIRST OPAQUE COATING

The first layer always consists of a white opaque wash serving as a neutral base. It is never modified. Saturate the powder with modeling fluid without rubbing the metal spatula against the glass plate. Crush the mixture with a pestle to refine it and improve its flow characteristics (Fig 2–1). Pick it up with the whole side of the opaque brush (Fig 2–2). Speed is critical, and the opaque must be kept moist throughout its whole application. Even though the modeling fluid delays drying, thin sections are more vulnerable to dehydration.

Follow a methodical sequence, starting with concave zones and using them as reservoirs; next, pull the opaque toward the incisal region to avoid thickening. For maxillary central incisors, coat the whole cervical periphery with fast, pulsing, overlapping motions (Fig 2–3). Next spread the coating by pulling and

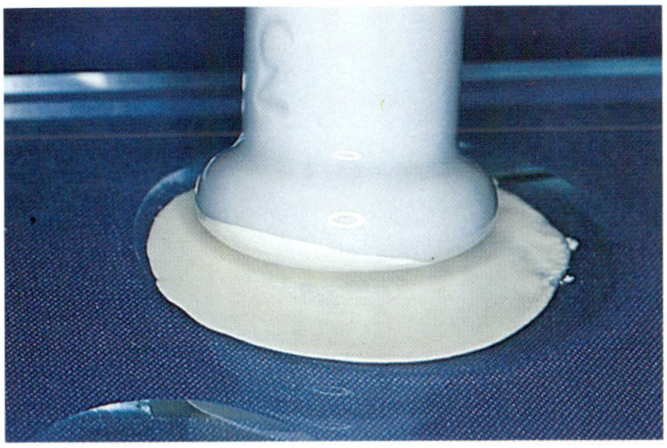

FIG 2–1

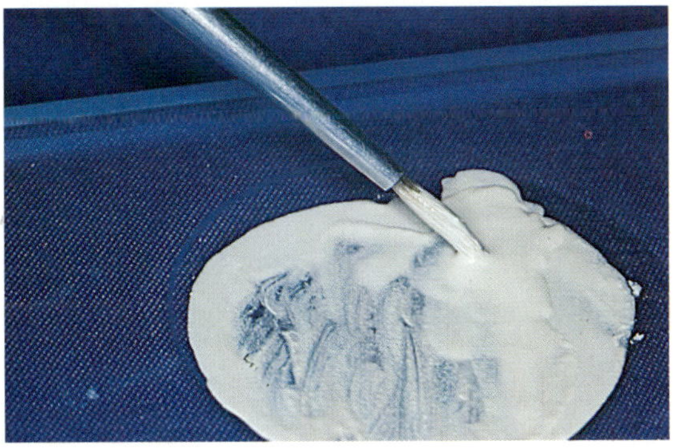

FIG 2–2

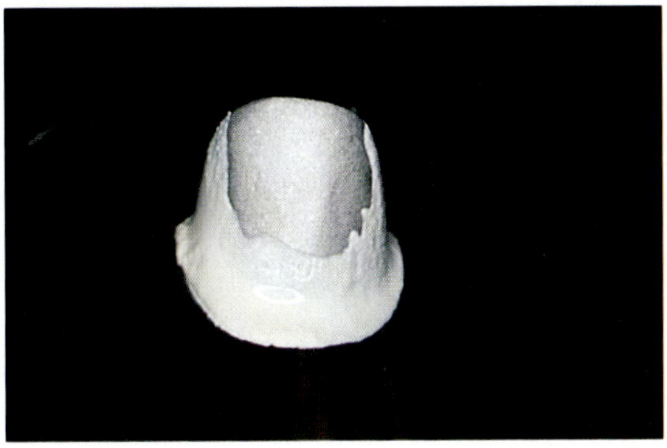

FIG 2–3

dragging it along the axial walls up to the incisal edge of the metal coping (Fig 2–4). For maxillary first molars, coat the whole cervical periphery and the axial walls (Fig 2–5). The occlusal surface is always started from the fossa so that the opaque may be spread to each occlusal tip (Fig 2–6).

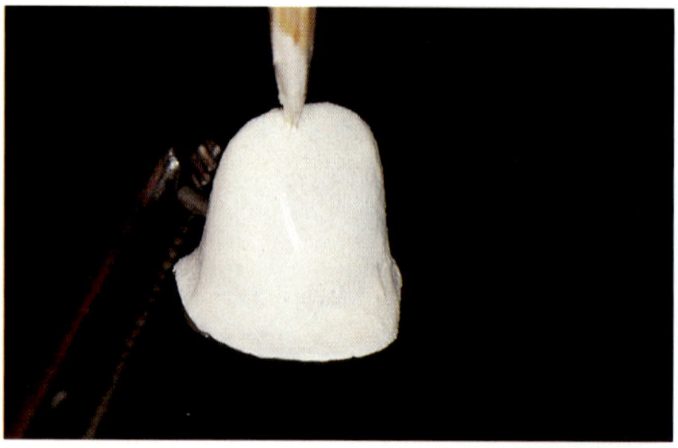

FIG 2–4

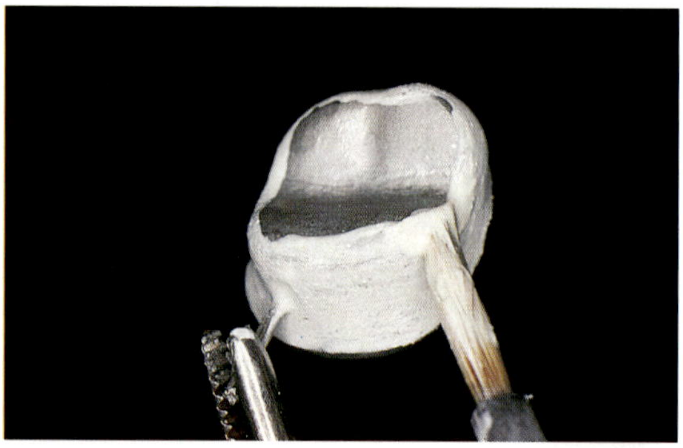

FIG 2–5

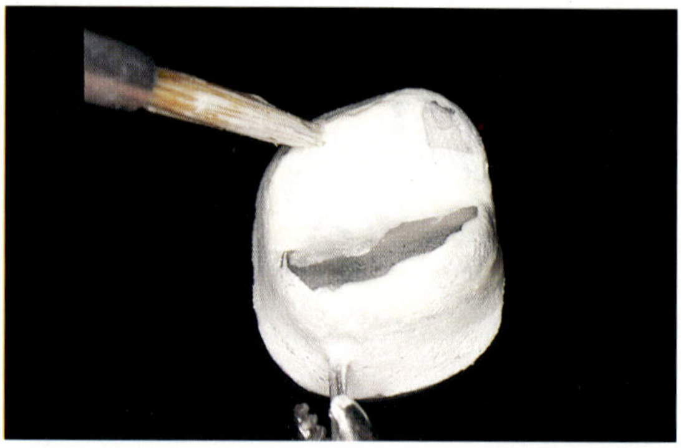

FIG 2–6

Apply two separate ultrasonic vibrations of 1 second each to bring the coating into more intimate contact with the metal. At this stage, there is no thickening; grayer zones will be covered in the next application. Fire according to the manufacturer's recommendation. The first opaque is fired in Figure 2–7.

SECOND OPAQUE COATING

The second coating is selected according to the prescribed shade and is generally unmodified. It is applied in adherence with the previous principles. Coating of the maxillary first molar follows exactly the sequence enumerated previously.

Coating of the maxillary central incisor is begun from the cervical periphery. The incisal tip must be covered separately and is continued with the proximal zones down to the cervix (Fig 2–8). Next, the axial walls are filled within this

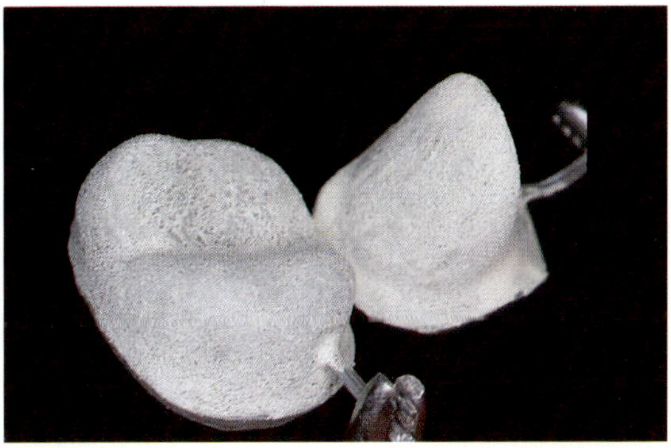

FIG 2–7

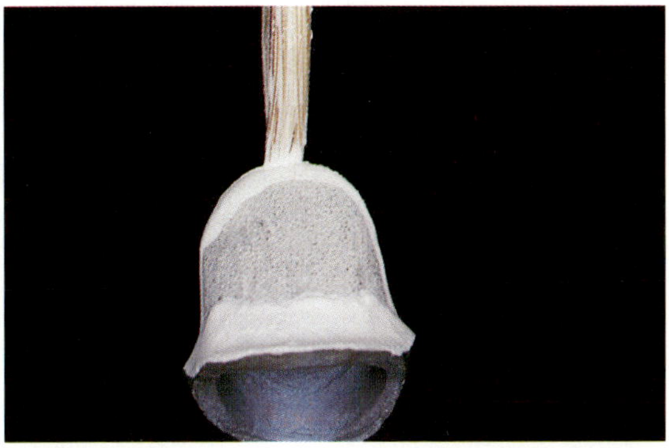

FIG 2–8

frame using fast sweeping strokes (Fig 2–9). This different progression prevents thickening of the opaque at the incisal tip.

Apply two separate ultrasonic vibrations of 1-second each to bring the mixture into more intimate contact with the fired layer. This uniform extra-thin opaque is now ready for firing. A three-unit bridge after opaquing is illustrated in Figure 2–10. In this sagittal section through a ceramic metal crown, the opaque layer is kept as thin as possible (Fig 2–11).

MODIFICATIONS OF OPAQUE

When the second opaque needs to be altered with modifiers, they must be directly applied onto the first fired wash; these modifiers substitute for the unmodified second opaque wherever they are applied. This maintains minimum thickness.

Modifications of opaque may be indicated when porcelain thickness is minimum, its brightness needs to be lowered through strong internal characterization, or depth and saturation need more emphasis. As a general rule the

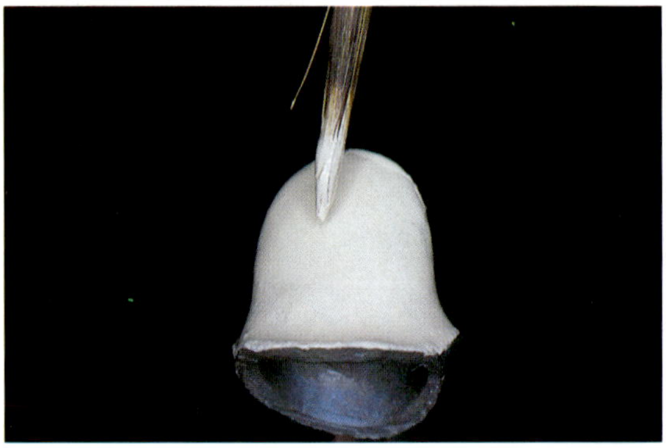

FIG 2–9

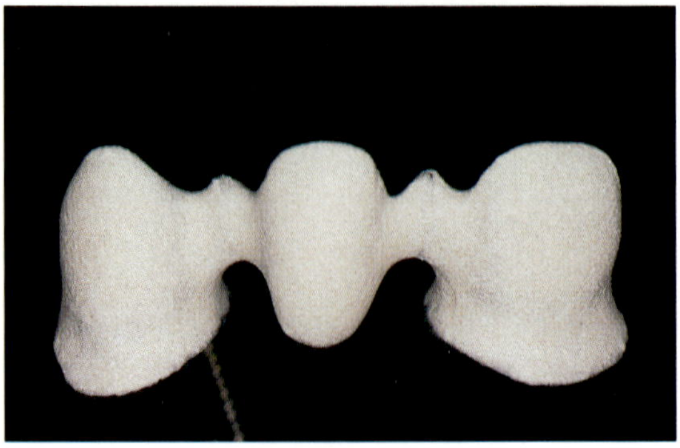

FIG 2–10

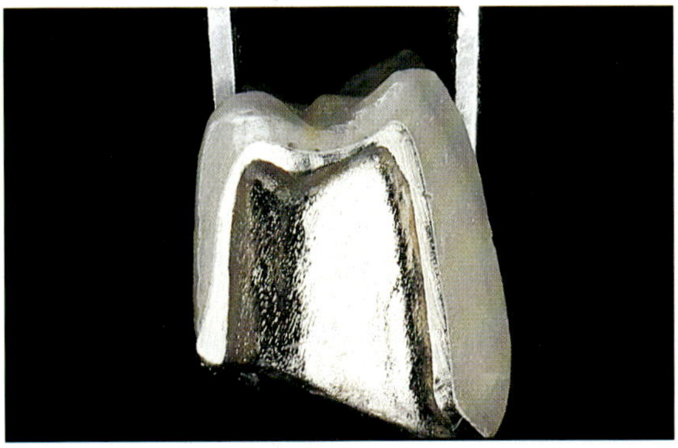

FIG 2–11

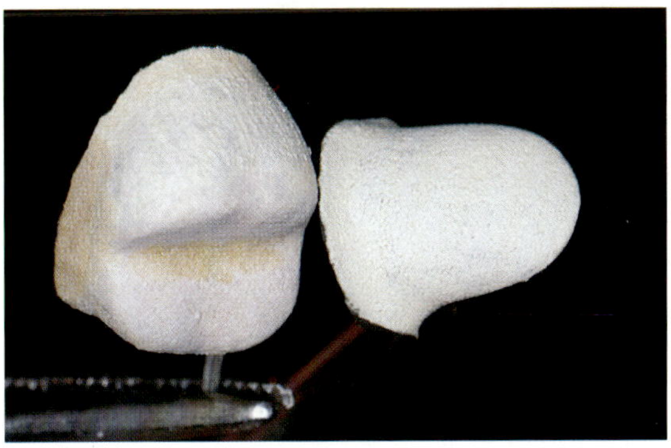

FIG 2–12

deeper the modification, the less prominent its effect on the overall color. With ideal dentin and enamel thickness, opaque modification is beneficial only at the cervical edge. (Indirect gold ceramic modification techniques[3] are sometimes preferred there, and are shown later.) Avoid excessive internal coloring; it may prove too strong and may spoil the final shade. Internal modification is a combination process in which deep subtle change still leaves room for further superficial alteration. In Figure 2–12, a typical correction (highlighted here with brightly colored tags) is depicted when occlusal and cervical thicknesses are critical. In the cervical area, orange opaque modifier (yellow tag) accentuates depth and saturation. In the proximal cervical zone, orange-brown opaque modifier (orange tag) accentuates depth.

The occlusal surface is coated with a mixture of pink and violet opaque modifiers to accentuate the illusion of elevation at the cusp tips; orange opaque modifier to accentuate the illusion of depth. After firing, the value is considerably lowered, and the colored effects are strong compared with the unmodified central.

REFERENCES

1. Barghi N, Lorenzana RE: Optimum thicknesses of opaque and body porcelain. *J. Prosthet Dent* 1982; 48:429.
2. McLean JW: *The Science and Art of Dental Ceramics*. Chicago, Quintessence Publishing Co, 1980, vol 2.
3. Yamamoto M: *Metal Ceramics*. Chicago, Quintessence Publishing Co, 1985.

Chapter 3

Principles of Buildup and Condensation

Both buildup and condensation are inseparable since they are conducted virtually simultaneously.

Condensation is the process by which unfired porcelain particles are packed together. Translucency of the fired crown (not considering its maturity) is directly related to the residual air bubble content. Satisfactory condensation of the buildup is achieved when the powder particles are as densely packed as possible, with all interstitial spaces filled with liquid binder only.[1] Maximum packing density promotes translucency and minimizes firing shrinkage. Air spaces produced in the unfired porcelain through mechanical entrapment or premature drying adversely affect translucency because their elimination is impossible with vacuum firing.[1] Several factors contribute to the increased porosity of the unfired porcelain:

1. Insufficient saturation of the mix
2. Overstirring of the powder in the liquid binder
3. Addition of too large amounts at once
4. Dehydration and frequent remoistening
5. Addition to an already dried zone

MOISTURE CONTROL

Initially paper tissue is used as a support to control the axial direction of the buildup and also serves to absorb excess moisture. As construction proceeds, it is essential to preserve distinct boundaries between the different colors to increase light refraction within the crown after firing. Excessive vibration causes distortion, blurring of the surface details, and especially interdiffusion between layers. Only short, low-amplitude vibrations (ultrasonic vibrations) may be effective at some specific stages. In fact, moisture control and, consequently, translucency rely on building techniques, sequencing, and working time.

Moisture Control Through Building Technique.— A brush is always preferred to a spatula because its body acts as a water reservoir, maintaining fluid balance through the porcelain bead. Its tip must be constantly moved in vibrating, tapping motions. These activate water at the surface of the unfired porcelain and facilitate addition of the bead (Fig 3-1). Never use any other type of vibration during the incremental buildup itself. A fine sable-hair brush provides for good water retention when very fine amounts need to be blended with the porcelain body. The versatility of the incremental brush technique is combined with surface tension phenomenon to create lobes and grooves from their associations. The most delicate configurations are best achieved with skillful mastery of the brush.[1]

Moisture Control Through Buildup Sequencing.— The likelihood of air entrapment is increased with large additions. Instead, start at the cervix (Fig 3-2),

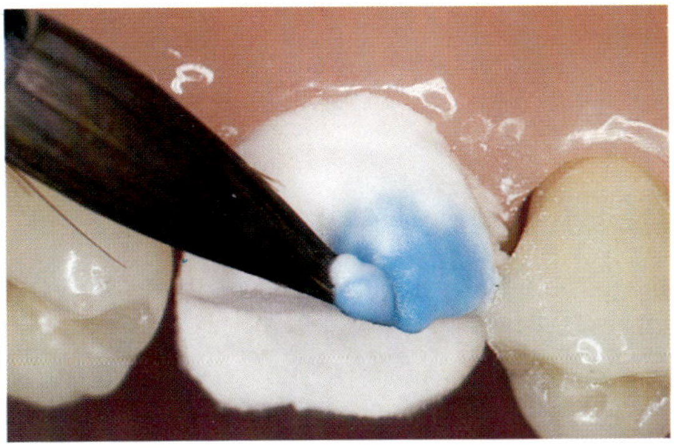

FIG 3–1

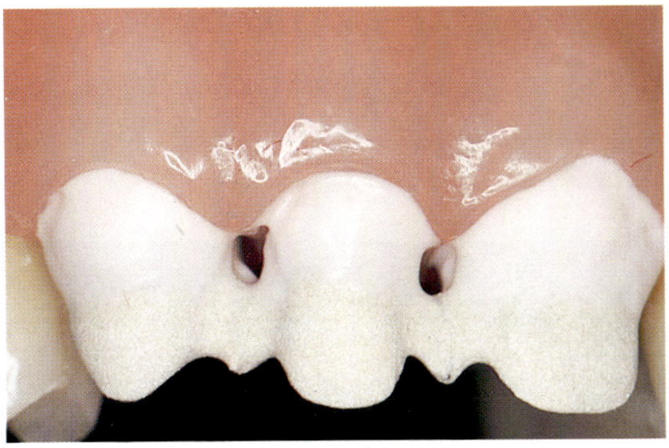

FIG 3–2

and use it as a base from which to erect a supporting structure (Fig 3-3). Additions proceed alongside and between the lobes, eventually filling in the whole surface. In this network approach, moisture is constantly available for each new application, which, in turn, blends quite easily to the wet mass.

When the construction must proceed to an altogether different area, it is directed toward it through a progression of proximal and occlusal ridges until another trilobed support is erected by continuity (Fig 3-4). This longitudinal progression, which draws moisture by continuity, allows these lobes to be developed against one another until they reach the other aspect of the crown (Fig 3-5). In some instances, however, too many increments applied in a very short

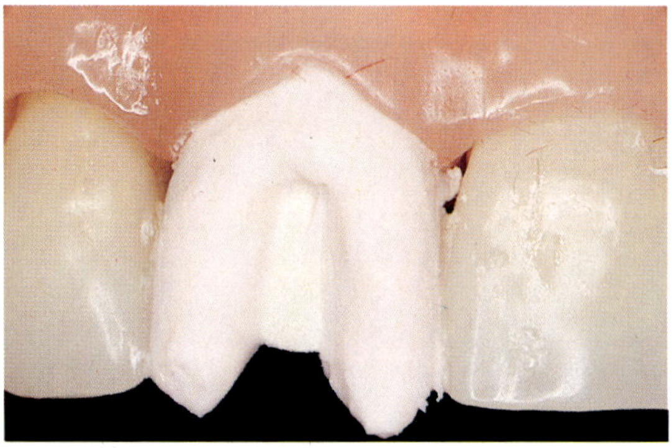

FIG 3–3

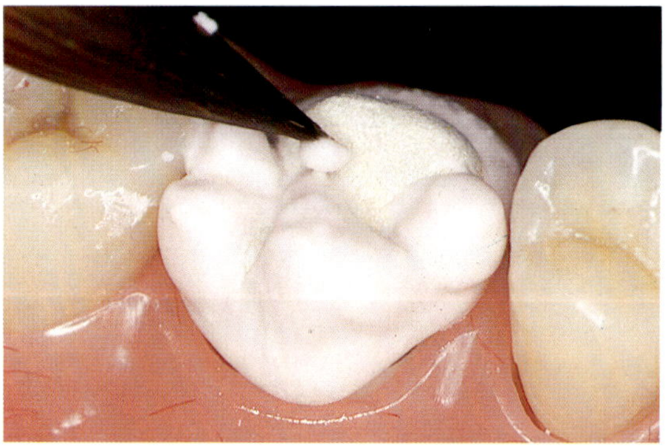

FIG 3–4

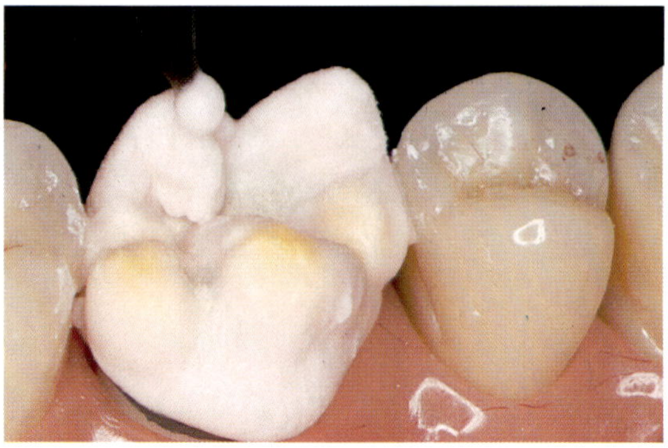

FIG 3–5

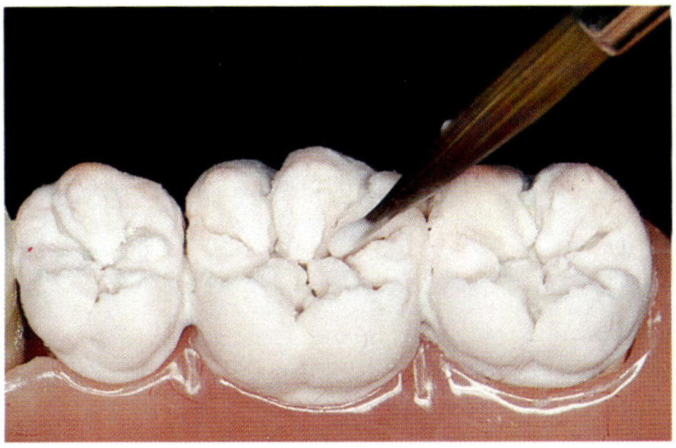

FIG 3–6

period of time may saturate the powder excessively with water, especially in the final stage of the occlusal construction, and contours may lose their sharpness. It is best to accomplish construction by proceeding back and forth, from one abutment to the next, until some evaporation takes place (Fig 3-6).

Moisture Control and Working Time.— Distilled water is the ideal liquid binder because it has no potential for leaving contaminating residues on burnout. In up to a three-unit bridge, the experienced ceramist can solely rely on working speed when building with distilled water and still avoid dehydration.

Beyond three units, working time needs to be prolonged since some constructions required up to 45 minutes. Add one part of modeling fluid to eight parts of distilled water. Besides extending significantly the working time, it preserves the plasticity of the buildup.

On completion of all constructions, water must still constitute 30% to 40% of the porcelain body weight.

REFERENCE

1. McLean JW: *The Art and Science of Dental Ceramics — A Collection of Monographs*. Louisiana State University School of Dentistry, Continuing Education Program, 1974.

Chapter **4**

Maxillary Central Incisor: One-Powder Construction

One-powder construction of the maxillary central incisor is the ideal starting exercise for incremental buildup. Adhere closely to all the fundamentals of buildup and condensation, and follow a logical sequence based on either network formation or longitudinal progression.

All constructions—whether complex or not—start with a fully contoured outline to provide for an accurate reference from which precise cutbacks and overlays are made possible.

Start on the labiocervical convexity and progress longitudinally around over the whole periphery (Fig 4–1).

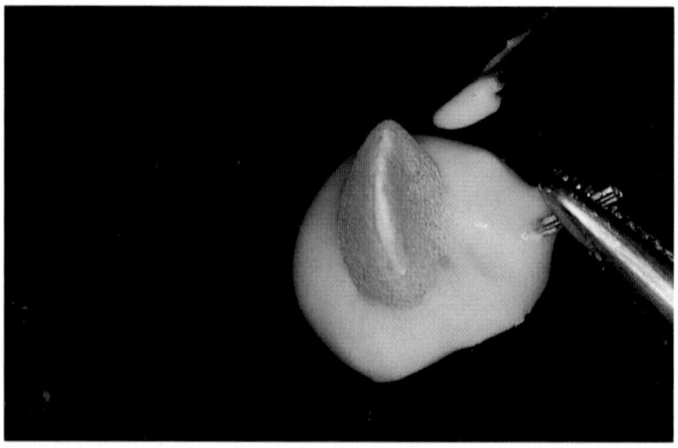

FIG 4–1

Erect each labial ridge separately (Fig 4–2); back them up with tissue paper for support and moisture control. The trilobed formation completes the labial network (Fig 4–3). It must already follow a typical triple convexity (Fig 4–4). The incisal edge is oversized in length only. Labiolingual contours are kept to normal dimensions.

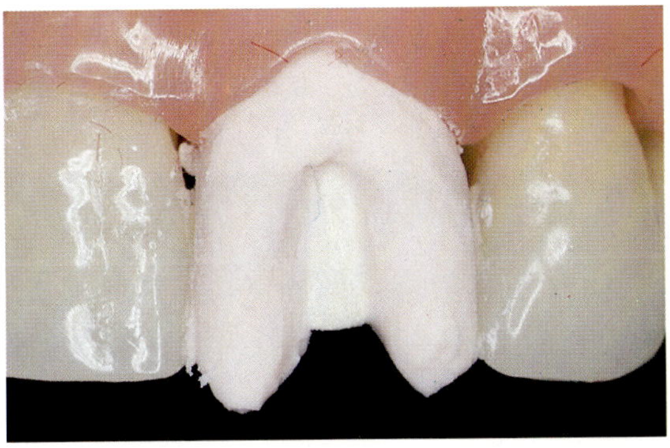

FIG 4–2

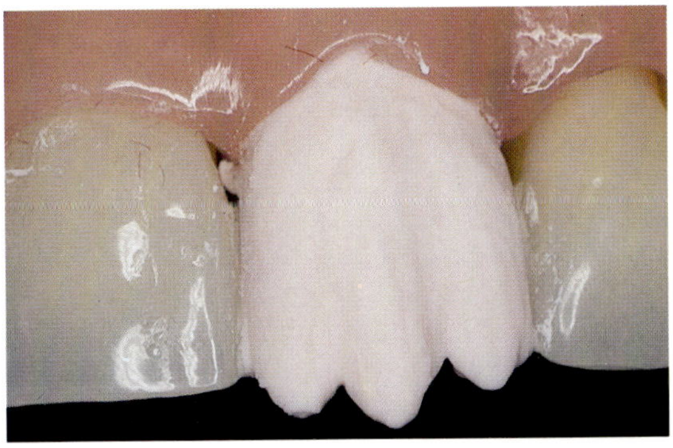

FIG 4–3

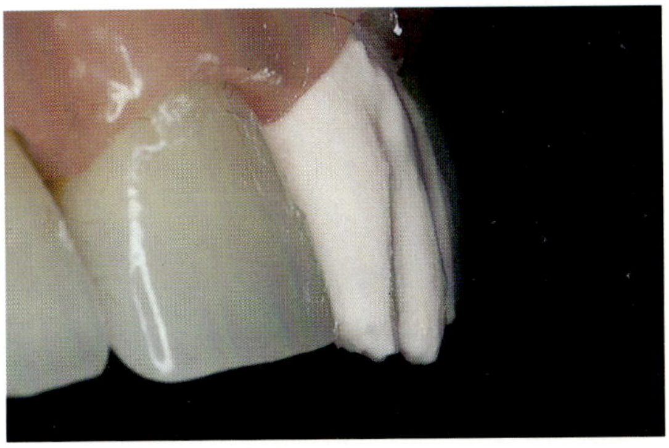

FIG 4–4

By continuity, carry each lingual marginal ridge from the incisal edge down to the cingulum area (Fig 4–5). Complete the lingual trilobe with a flat extension from the cingulum to the incisal edge. The lingual fossa is filled in between and along each lobe (Fig 4–6). Always delicately tap and vibrate the tip of the brush to activate moisture on the surface. Coat the mandibular incisors with disclosing color paste and (TANAKA Bite = X, Skokie, Ill.) and delicately, lightly tap the models into slight occlusion until very slight resistance is felt. The premature

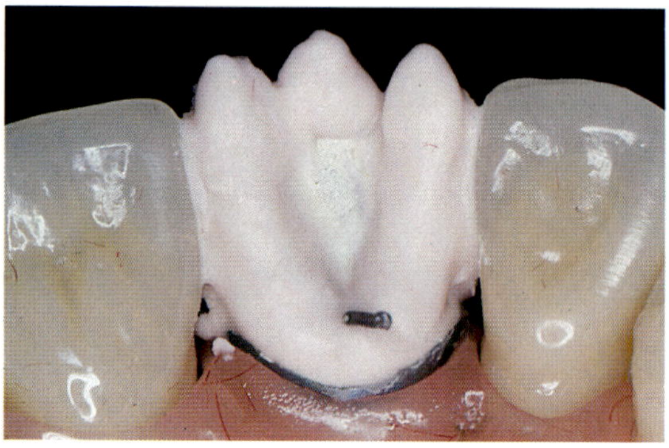

FIG 4–5

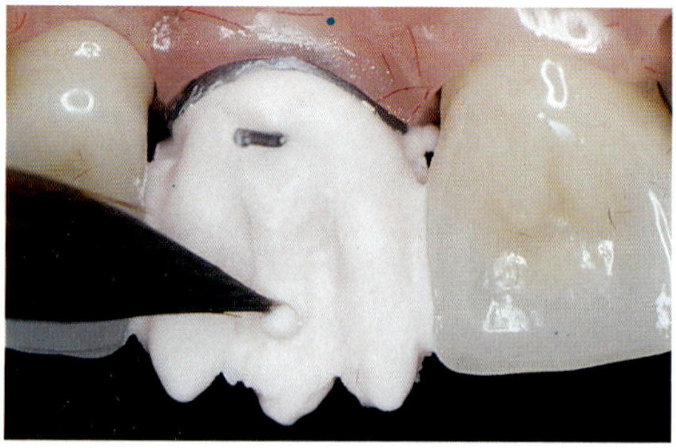

FIG 4–6

contacts will create some concavities. They are rounded with the tip of the brush. Repeat the same process until harmonious occlusion is achieved (Fig 4–7). The labial outline is completed between and along each lobe (Fig 4–8). Preserve the convexity of the labial marginal ridges. Shave any excess with the carving blade in light sweeping motions to refine and polish the labial contour (Fig 4–9).

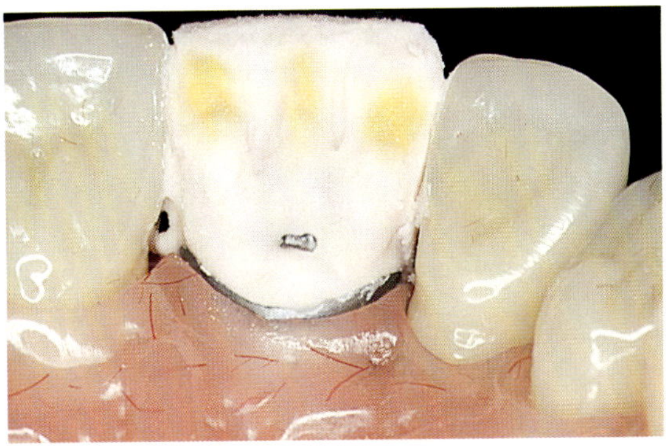

FIG 4–7

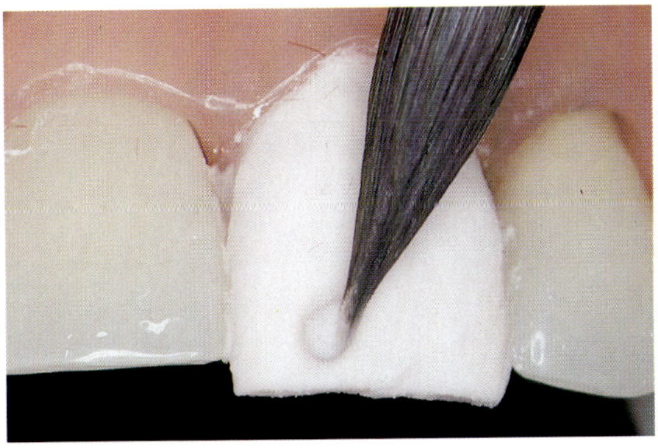

FIG 4–8

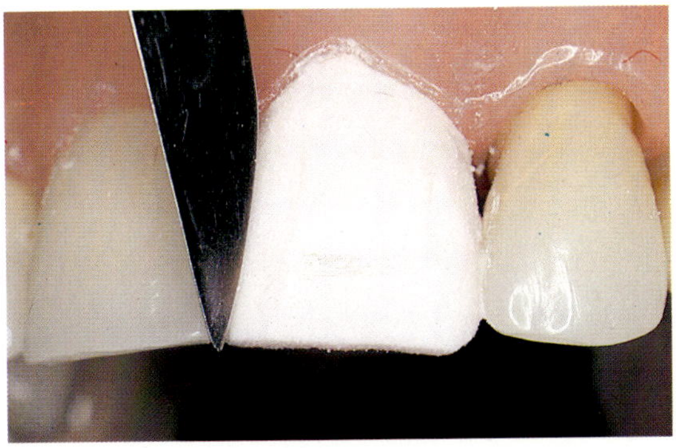

FIG 4–9

The large soft-hair brush is pressed in cervicoincisal strokes only. Stronger pressure on the incisal edge draws it inward to conform to the adjacent central incisor (Fig 4–10). To gain better judgment, carve the incisal edge to the same length as the adjacent tooth in this exercise only (Fig 4–11).

Apply two separate ultrasonic vibrations of 1 second each. Follow each one with an application of tissue paper for elimination of excess moisture.

At the end of this exercise there should be no premature drying, and all interstitial spaces should be filled with distilled water only. Further cutbacks and overlays are possible without any remoistening (Fig 4–12).

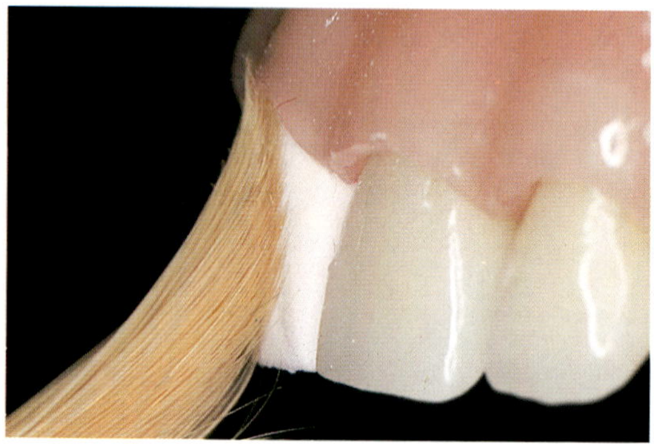

FIG 4–10

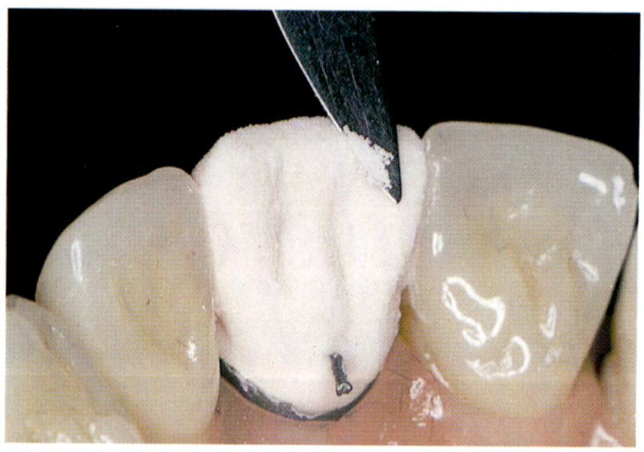

FIG 4–11

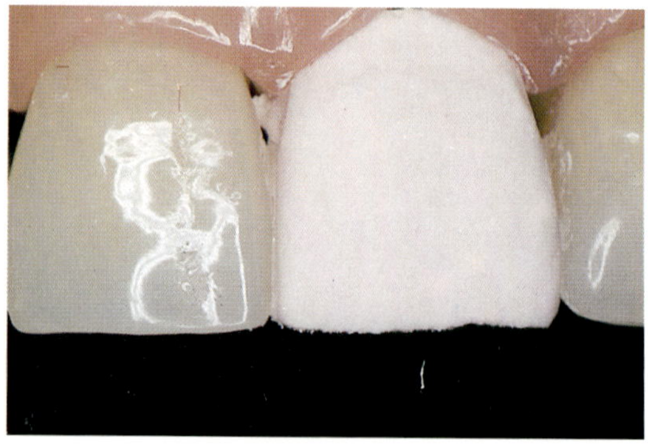

FIG 4–12

Chapter **5**

Maxillary First Molar: One-Powder Construction

This exercise is a methodic buildup based on two networks connected with a progression through the proximal marginal ridges.

The complete cervical periphery serves as the base of the construction (Fig 5–1). Erect each lingual cusp lobe from a cervical to an incisal direction (Fig 5–

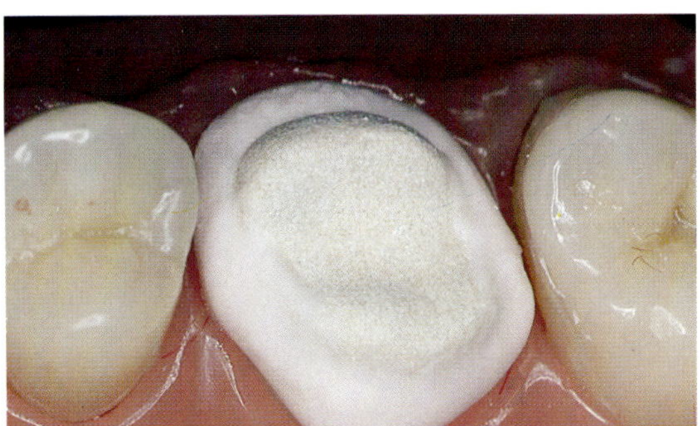

FIG 5–1

2). The outline of the lingual groove is automatically created at their junction.

Dry off excess water on each lobe. This adds some rigidity and support before the next additions are made.

Extend from each cusp a proximal marginal lobe and a lingual triangular ridge (Fig 5–3). Coat the opposing dentition with disclosing color paste, and

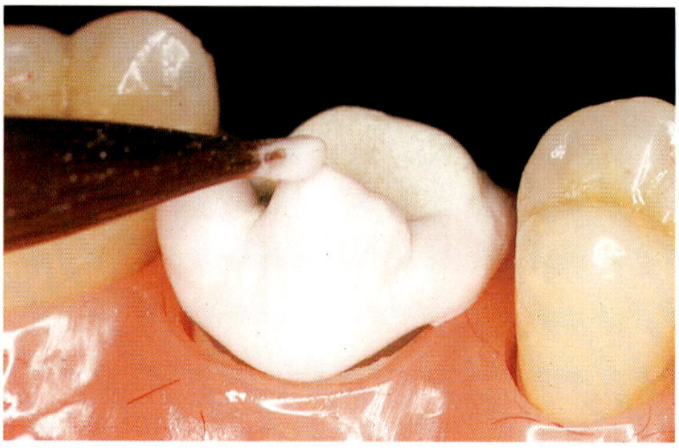

FIG 5–2

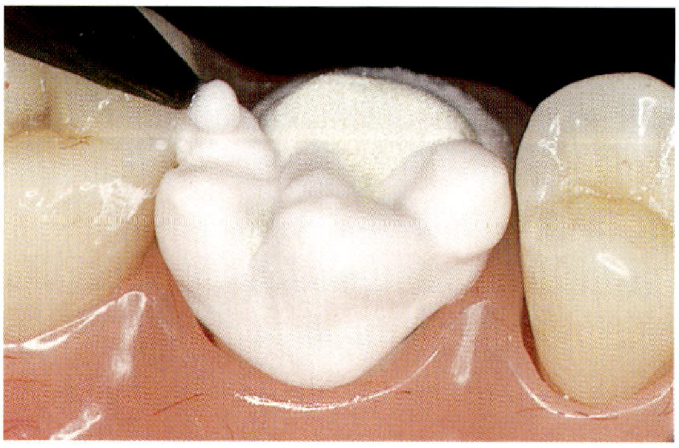

FIG 5–3

delicately bring the models into light occlusion until slight resistance is felt. It may be necessary to realign a whole cusp tip with the opposing fossa. There is enough plasticity in the buildup to displace it with controlled pressure of the brush. Adjust the occlusion until four centric areas are properly located (Fig 5–4). This completes the lingual outline. The labial cusp ridges are constructed as extensions of the proximal marginal ridges (Fig 5–5).

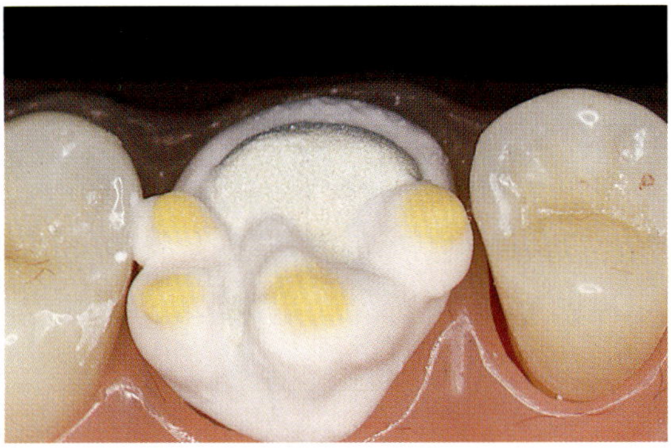

FIG 5–4

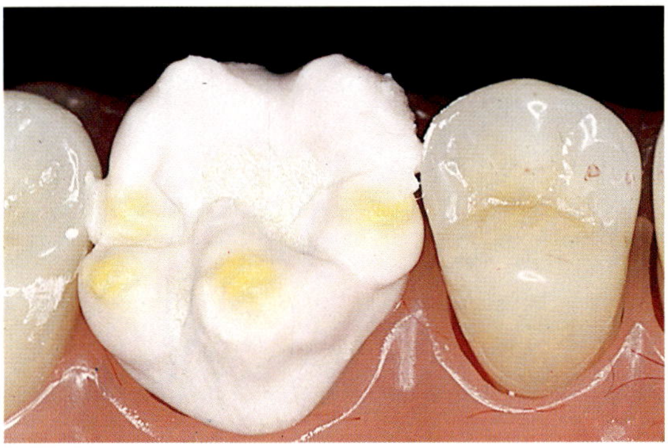

FIG 5–5

Connect each cusp tip to the cervical base (Fig 5–6), and fill in and along the labial network (Fig 5–7). Complete the labial anatomy with the buildup brush and the large soft-hair brush only (Fig 5–8).

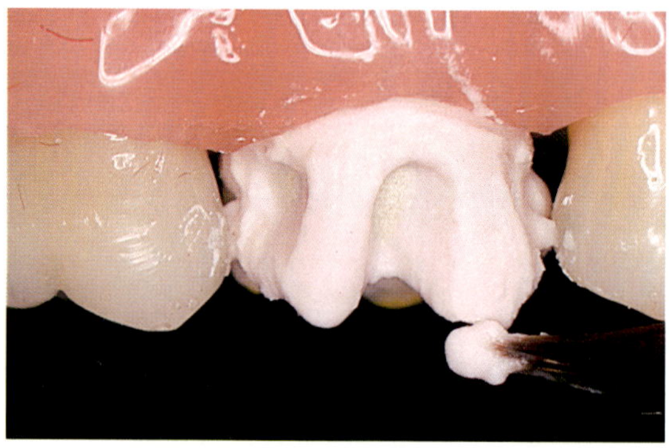

FIG 5–6

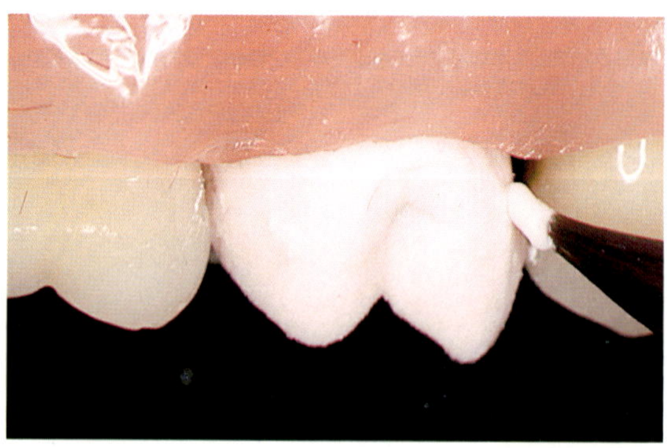

FIG 5–7

The triangular ridges are laid at the inner aspect of the labial cusps. The occlusal groove pattern results from the junction of all the convexities (Fig 5–9). Recheck the occlusion, and place the final additions with the fine sable brush (Fig 5–10). Use its tip to emphasize the primary and supplemental grooves.

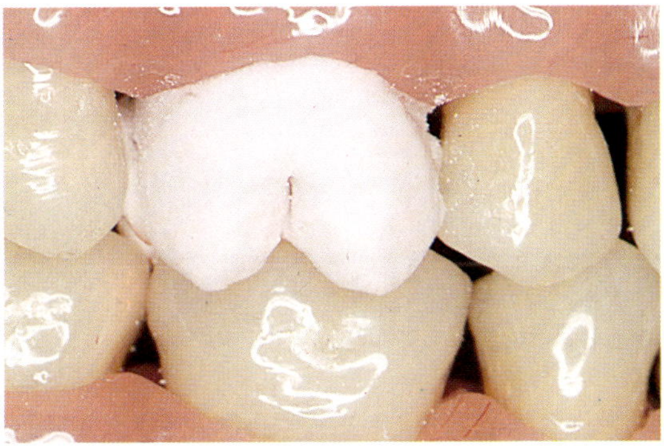

FIG 5–8

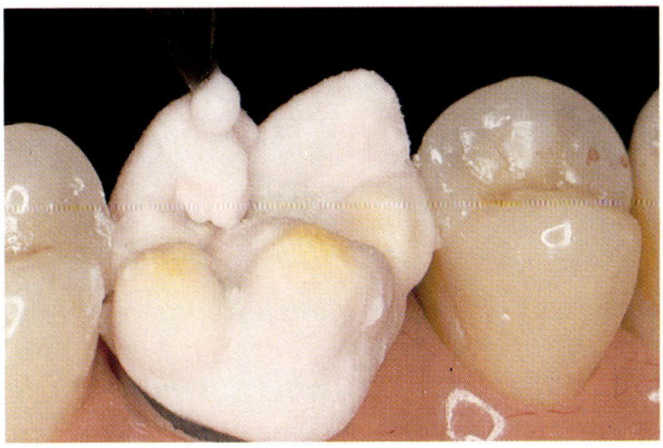

FIG 5–9

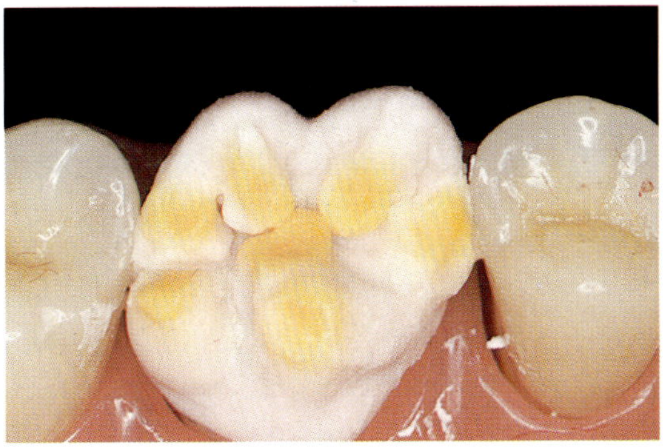

FIG 5–10

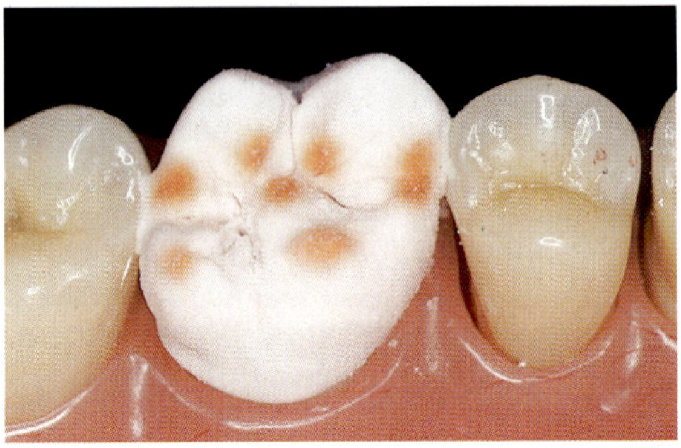

FIG 5–11

Refine the lingual surface, and polish the final anatomy with the large soft-hair brush. The whole buildup is constructed to full normal contours at the vertical dimension of occlusion with the brush only. As explained before, moisture control is facilitated with this sequence (Fig 5–11).

Apply two separate ultrasonic vibrations of 1-second each. Dry off the excess moisture.

At the end of this exercise there should be no premature drying. All interstitial spaces are filled with distilled water only. Further cutbacks and overlays are performed without any remoistening.

Chapter 6

Maxillary Three-Unit Bridge: One-Powder Construction

All anatomical contours are built to exact dimensions except for the incisal edges, which are oversized. As soon as the initial labial outlines are developed, they must conform to a triple convexity. Each labial lobe progresses lingually to create a lingual ridge and flow into the cingulum region.

Start condensing at the cervical periphery of the central incisor. Progress to the lateral incisor and last to the canine (Fig 6–1). The central incisor is completed

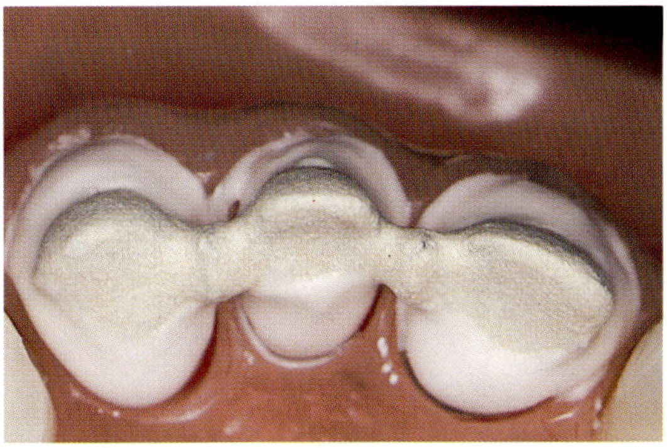

FIG 6–1

first, duplicating the sequence described in Chapter 4 (Fig 6–2).

The lateral incisor is constructed next according to the same principles, but only two labial and lingual ridges are formed (Fig 6–3). The mesial marginal ridge is accentuated to create slight rotation and individuality (Fig 6–4). Its labial aspect should be more rounded than the central.

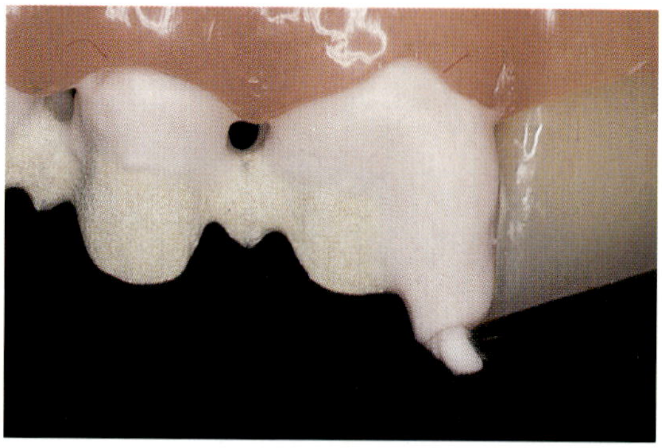

FIG 6–2

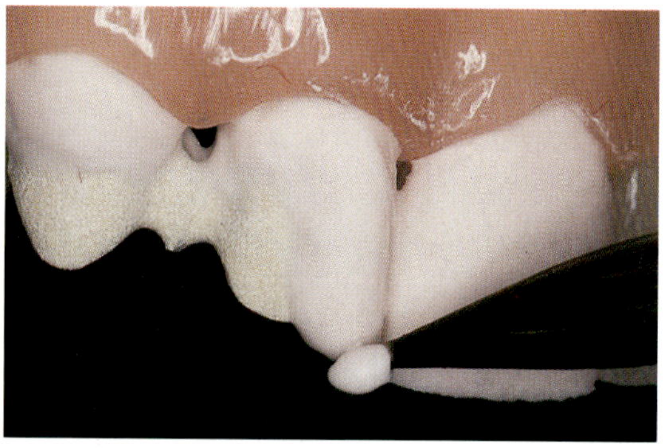

FIG 6–3

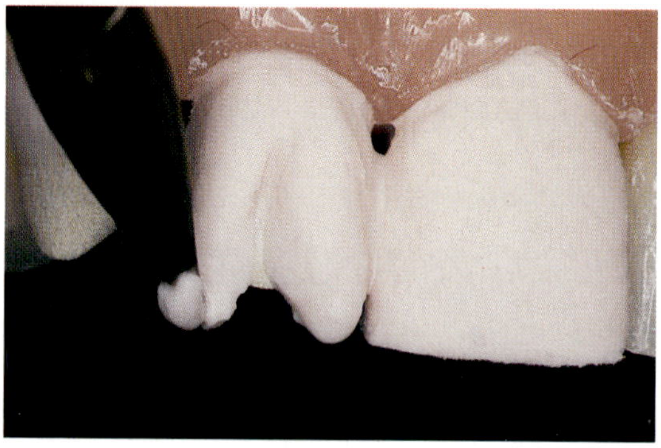

FIG 6–4

The canine follows the same building progression, but its labial and lingual median ridges are more accentuated (Fig 6–5). The whole mesial labial portion of the tooth is convex, whereas the distal cervical part is concave.

Adjust the occlusion with the buildup brush and a Roach carver (Fig 6–6).

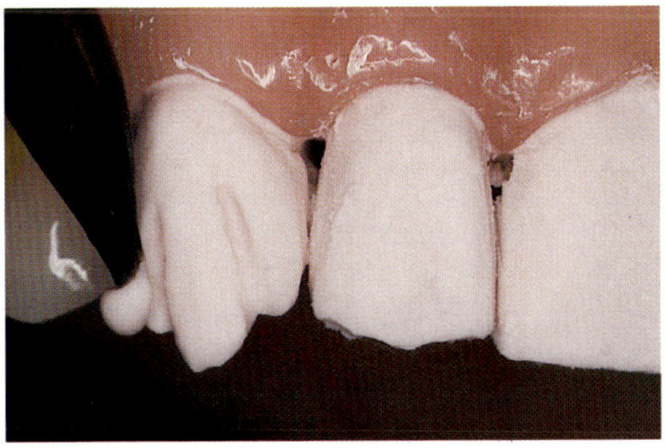

FIG 6 5

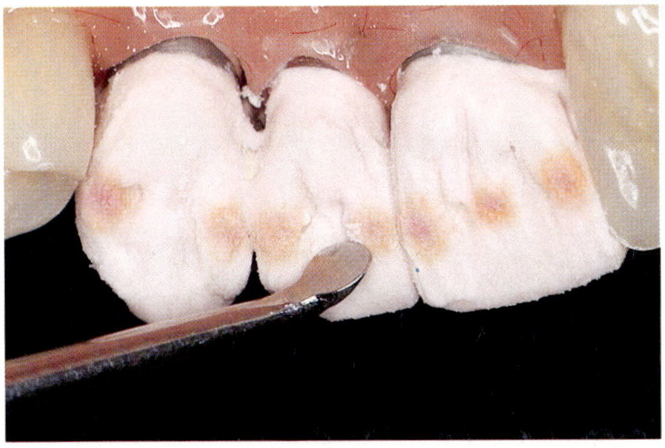

FIG 6–6

Do not slide the models in protrusive and lateral excursions; this may break and detach the unfired porcelain from the underlying opaque. Instead, extrapolate the lingual contour by gently tapping the models along two to three distinct portions of the excursive pathways.

Plan for occlusal refinement after each firing. Apply two separate ultrasonic vibrations of 1 second each, and dry off the excess distilled water. The completed dentin buildup is shown in Figure 6–7.

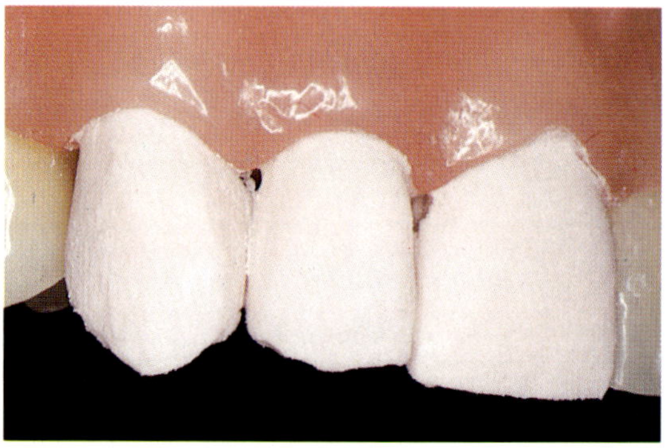

FIG 6–7

Chapter 7

Mandibular Three-Unit Bridge: One-Powder Construction

The axial and occlusal anatomy will be built to full contours in maximum intercuspation.

Form each labial convexity so that it chamfers into the opaque layer (Fig 7–1). Proceed in the same fashion to the lingual cervical areas.

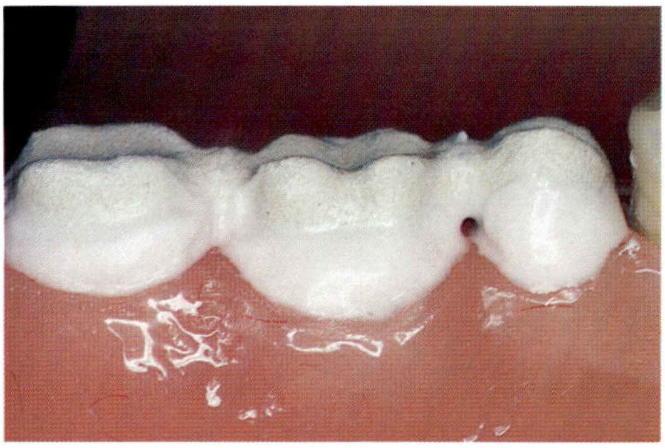

FIG 7–1

Develop the buccal cusp cone from the cervical base (Fig 7–2). The cusp tip is adjusted in length and aligned buccolingually until it contacts the opposing fossa. Form the buccal line angles from the cervical base (Fig 7–3). Repeat the same procedure with, respectively, one and two additional lobes for the second and first molars. The labial developmental grooves are automatically created at

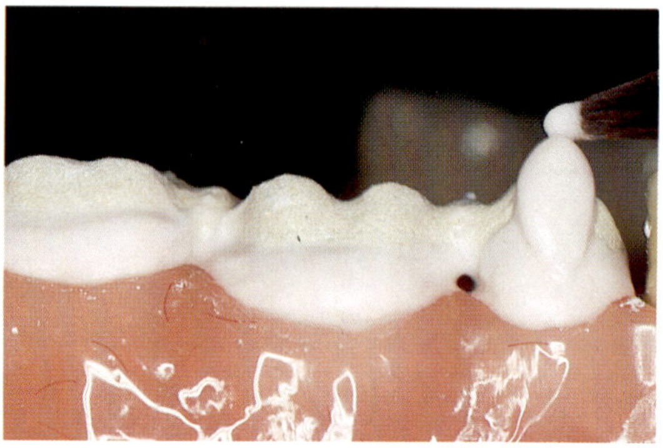

FIG 7–2

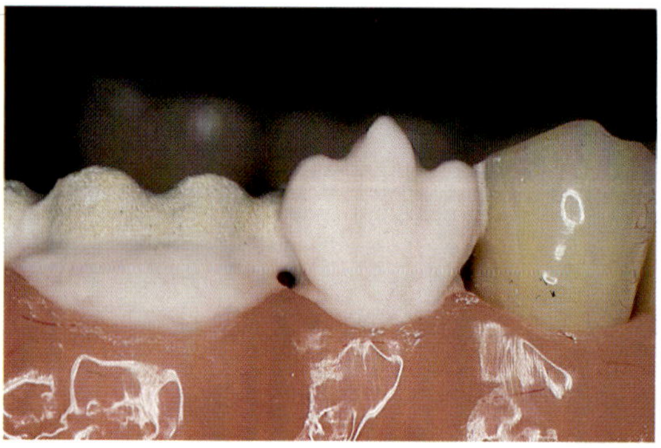

FIG 7–3

their junction (Fig 7–4). Examine the position of every lobe (Fig 7–5). There is enough plasticity in the buildup to press every cusp tip into a better alignment with the opposing fossa or embrasure if necessary. Dry excess moisture off. This adds rigidity to each cone. The marginal ridges extend from the mesial and distal cusp ridges (Fig 7–6). Triangular ridges descend from the cusp tip toward the

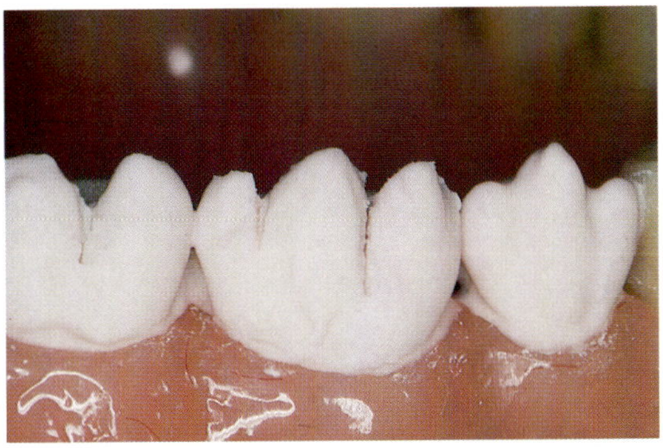

FIG 7–4

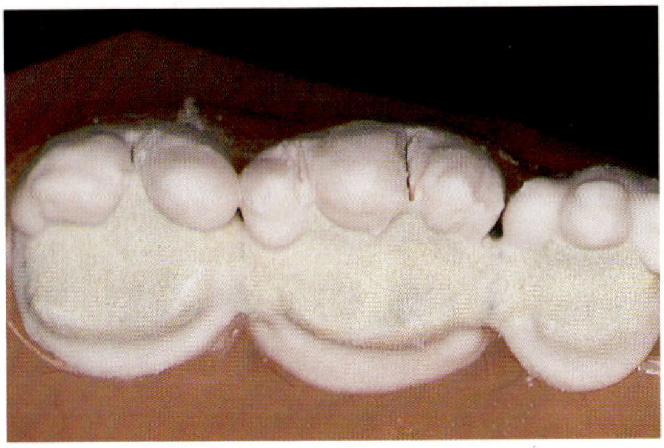

FIG 7–5

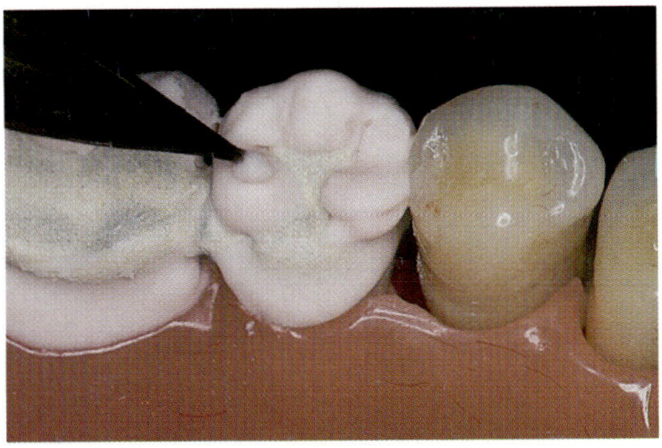

FIG 7–6

center of the occlusal surface (Fig 7–7). Adjust the occlusal prematurities with the buildup brush and the Roach carver (Fig 7–8).

Form two cusp cones from every linguocervical base. Fill in and along each lobe with small increments to complete the linguoaxial walls (Fig 7–9). Bring

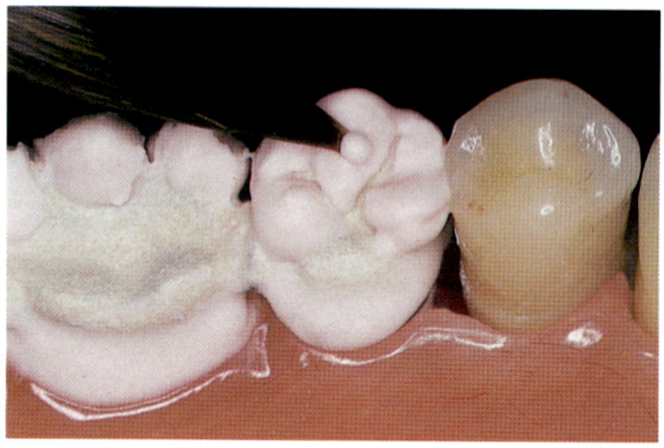

FIG 7–7

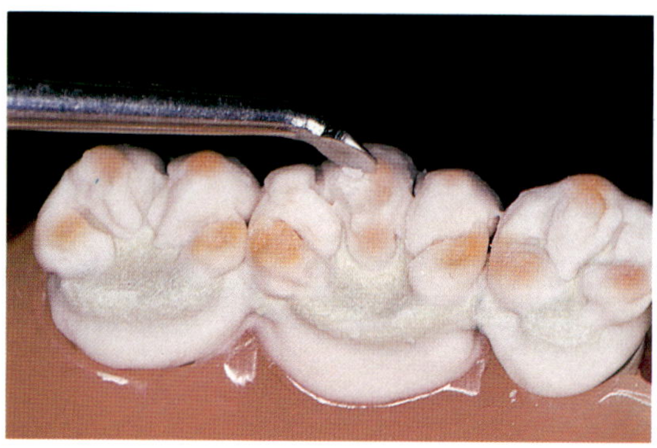

FIG 7–8

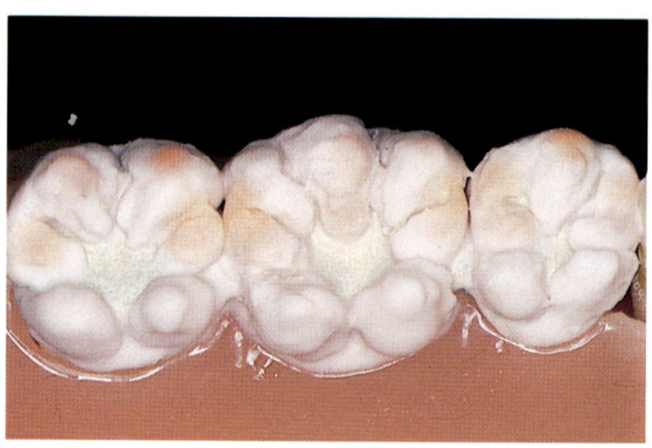

FIG 7–9

the lingual triangular ridges from the cusp tips until they contact the inner buccal inclines. Finish the axial contours with the large soft-hair brush (Fig 7–10).

All occlusal additions and corrections are now made with very fine wet beads (Fig 7–11). This is the most delicate part since the porcelain powder may become excessively saturated with water, and sharp details may be lost.

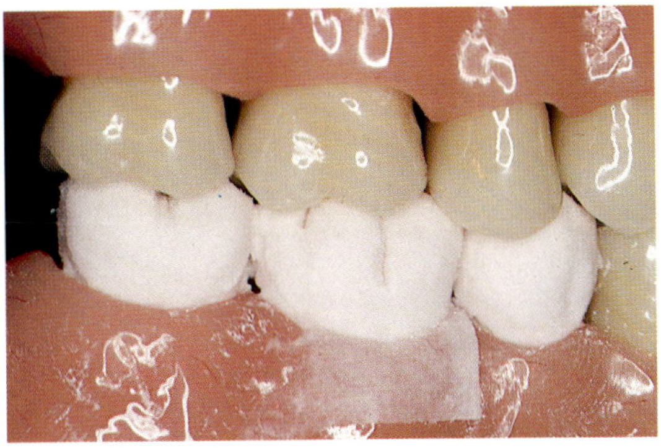

FIG 7–10

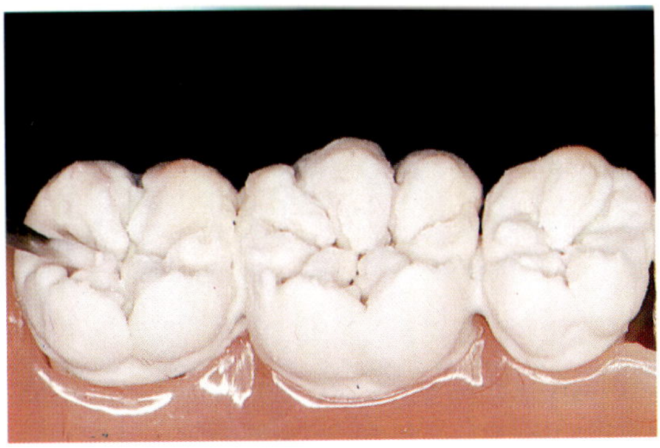

FIG 7–11

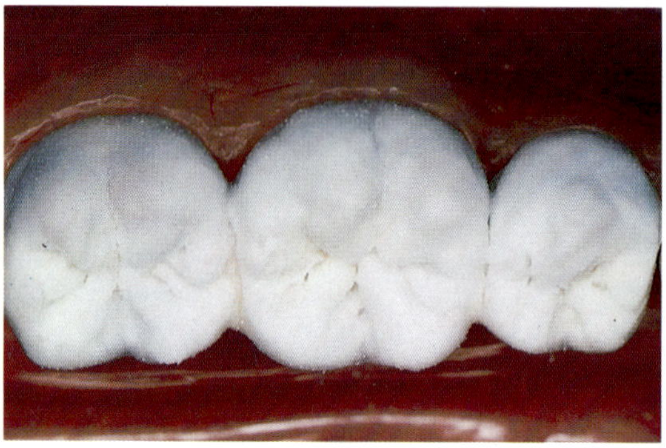

FIG 7–12

Spread the additions back and forth from one tooth to the next so that enough evaporation takes place.

Manipulate the fine sable brush very precisely; it directs accessory lobes and deepens supplemental grooves. It adds and carves as dictated by occlusal and anatomical specifications. Do not use any carving blade. The most exquisite details can be reproduced only with the brush technique. Major lateral interferences are carefully eliminated without breaking or detaching the unfired porcelain from the underlying opaque. Plan for occlusal adjustments after each firing.

On completion, apply two separate ultrasonic vibrations of 1 second each, and dry off the excess distilled water binder (Fig 7–12).

Chapter 8

Translucency and Firing

One of the most difficult objectives of the dental ceramist is to obtain and preserve translucency. Firing in the oven must be carefully controlled so that the benefits of good condensation may be maintained.

Avoid contamination of the oven with flux and metal vapors residues, which eventually coat the walls of the muffle chamber. Post ceramic soldering must be altogether performed in a separate furnace. Silver alloys are not recommended as long as they have potential for greening porcelain. Distilled water is the ideal liquid binder since it leaves no residue on burnout. When working time needs to be extended, opaque liquid is mixed with distilled water in the ratio of 1:8 with dentin powder only. The enamel and transparent powder are always exclusively mixed with distilled water. Similarly, surface colorants are always mixed with 1 part of stain liquid to 10 parts of distilled water to minimize the potential for residual contaminant.

A very active oven yields better heat radiancy and deeper heat penetration over time than if it were used infrequently. Better results are even often produced at the end of a busy day after numerous firings. It is strongly recommended to run at least three continuous firing cycles in the morning with an empty muffle chamber before the first crown is fired.

Heat distribution inside the furnace should be as uniform as possible. However, it is as critical to dispose each unit back in the same exact position and over the same firing tray during every cycle. It might otherwise be subjected to a different temperature if it were placed at a different level of the chamber every time.

Heat penetration inside the porcelain must reach the deepest layers. The firing temperature must be raised by 5° to 10°C for a bridge according to its bulk and the number of units. Similarly, elimination of the liquid binder must be complete especially in the deepest aspect, which is the most porous,[1] and predrying time must be adjusted from 4 minutes for a single unit up to 9 minutes for a long span bridge. When a second body firing is indicated, predrying time is reduced to 2 minutes, since new additions are comparatively smaller.

Modern furnaces with improved temperature monitors represent significant progress, but regardless of any sophistication, the temperature gauge display may in time differ from the muffle temperature. Regular calibration must take place every 3 months. If the oven was not used for more than 1 week, run a purge cycle to eliminate any residual moisture.

Translucency depends on vacuum quality. It reduces residual air spaces in the porcelain so that it can shrink to the densest possible mass. Inspect the vacuum pump for any moisture infiltration, and check its pressure once yearly. When the vacuum pressure is intentionally reduced along the 740– to 760 mm range, it creates an opaque, dense porcelain with a sclerotic aspect.[2]

Voltage fluctuations may be caused by other electrical units in the laboratory. The power outlet of the oven should connect only to the central power supply independently of any other appliance.

Adhere to the manufacturer's instructions to avoid too rapid firing cycles. These result in uncompletely fired porcelain and increase residual porosity.

Longer vacuum timing than recommended may cause blistering. Firing to higher temperatures than necessary will produce devitrification and graying of the porcelain.

Slower firing cycles reduce the likelihood of entrapped residual air bubbles during shrinkage and consequently improve translucency as long as firing temperature is accordingly reduced to control maturity of the porcelain. The objective is to locate for that particular oven the rate of firing and temperature equilibrium that yields optimum translucency and sufficient maturity as allowed by the thermal compatibility of the alloy with the porcelain. For example, Crystar Porcelain (Unitek Company) fired to 940°C at 100°C/min can also be fired to 900°C at 50°C/minute.

When beautiful translucency is achieved on the first firing, the priority of the ceramist from then on is to preserve it through the second firing and the glazing. The fewer firings dental porcelain is subjected to, the less devitrification and cloudiness.[3] All single units must be completed with one body firing. All bridges should be completed within two body firings. The second firing temperature is lowered by 10°C to 20°C, with the firing rate reduced by 10°C to 15°C/minute.

Glazing also has influence over the maturity stage and should be conducted with a quick rise in temperature to the lowest possible temperature, so that only the most superficial layer is affected. Its effect is both time and temperature dependent. Time is determined according to the desired surface aspect. It is always performed without vacuum to prevent bubbling through the porcelain.

It is now evident that translucency depends on the interaction of several factors: (1) crown selection, (2) porosity in the unfired porcelain, (3) air elimination during sintering, and (4) prevention of devitrification.

Crown Selection.—When one is selecting between an aluminous jacket crown,[4] a bonded aluminous crown,[5] or a porcelain fused to metal crown, the benefits of bonding to metal in terms of tensile and flexural strength increase and surface defects reduction must be weighed against the decrease in light transmission through the crown. The increased opacity of high expansion porcelain is another consideration, but it is still possible to achieve depth of translucency with these by promoting internal light refraction and diffusion when sufficient thickness is provided.

Porosity in the Unfired Porcelain.—This is affected by the consistency of the mix, the buildup technique and its condensation, the buildup sequence, and the moisture control.

Air Elimination During Sintering.—This is a function of predrying time, heat penetration, firing temperature, and vacuum quality.

Prevention of Devitrification.—Partial fusion at the grain boundaries must be maintained after glazing. Rate of firing and firing temperature selection, number of body firings, glazing time and temperature, and temperature control accuracy are all essential.

REFERENCES

1. McLean JW: *The Art and Science of Dental Ceramics—A Collection of Monographs.* New Orleans, Louisiana State University School of Dentistry, Continuing Education Program, 1974.
2. Geller W: Personal communication, Paris, 1983.
3. McLean JW: *The Science and Art of Dental Ceramics.* Chicago, Quintessence Publishing Co, 1980, vol 2.
4. McLean JW, Hughes TH: The reinforcement of dental porcelain with ceramic oxides. *Br Dent J* 1965; 119:251–257.
5. McLean JW, Sced IR: The bonded alumina crown: The bonding of platinum to aluminous dental porcelain using tin oxyde coatings. *Aust Dent J* 1976; 21:2.

Chapter 9

Maxillary Central Incisor: Three-Powder Construction

The central incisor is first built to full contours in dentin to serve as a precise reference frame for the color additions. It is carved back to provide space for the enamel porcelain. The final translucent overlay compensates for firing shrinkage and creates additional depth of translucency. Sharp internal demarcation must be kept at all times between all three layers to emphasize light refraction within the crown after firing. Moisture control and adequate condensation are imperative.

The dentin buildup is constructed to full contours according to the complete sequence described in Chapter 4. The incisal edge is oversized by 1 mm (Fig 9–1). All other aspects are kept within normal dimensions except for the labio-

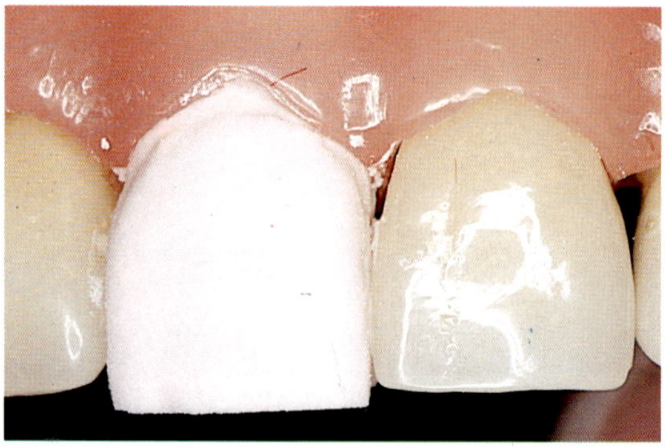

FIG 9–1

cervical convexity. It is slightly accentuated since it will neither be cut back nor overlaid and will still be subjected to some shrinkage.

The cutback allows for placement of the enamel porcelain. The amount of labial and proximal reduction is dictated by the shade prescription. In Figure 9–2, it is extended down to the middle third of the labial surface. The labial reduction consists in lateral beveling sweeps of the carving blade so that the dentin is feathered incisally with no abrupt delineation of the dentinoenamel blend line. In this fashion, the dentin background will fade progressively toward the incisal edge since it was already oversized by 1 mm. When mamelons are indicated, a fingered dentin background will create a sharper contrast against the enamel.

If the initial dentin buildup is not oversized incisally, the enamel will be allowed to extend without any dentin subsurface, and the incisal edge may contrast excessively with the rest of the tooth and appear grayer.

For softened individualization in the proximal region, dentin is progressively decreased at each extremity without breaking contact with the adjacent teeth and still allow for enamel wraparound (Fig 9–3). The dentin is probed to ensure

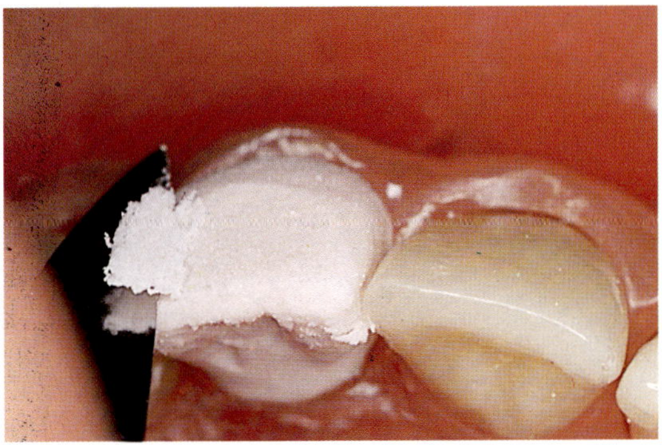

FIG 9–2

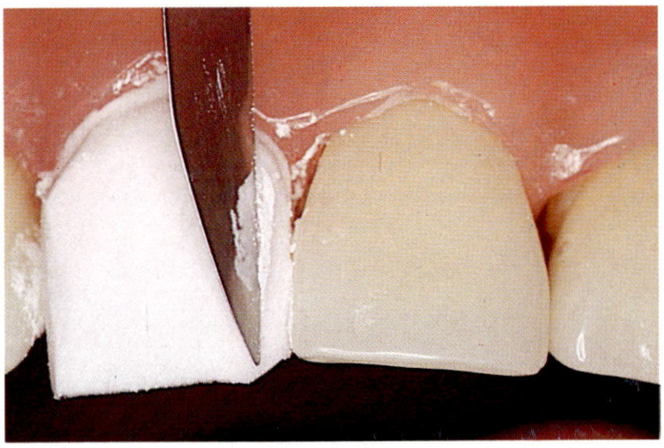

FIG 9–3

adequate thickness ranging from 0.6 to 0.8 mm (Fig 9–4). Thinner dentin results in higher value because of opaque proximity.

The enamel powder is mixed with distilled water and applied in small increments over the reduced aspects. Typical vibrations of the tip of the brush induce water onto the surface of the buildup. The enamel construction proceeds in a continuous sequence from distal to mesial until the labial aspect is restored back to normal contours with the incisal edge oversized by 1 mm (Fig 9–5). If a mamelon effect is desired, it is created in the dentin buildup before enamel construction (Fig 9–6).

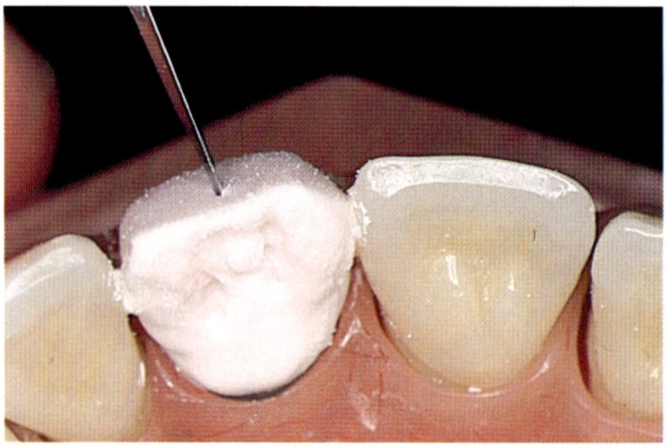

FIG 9–4

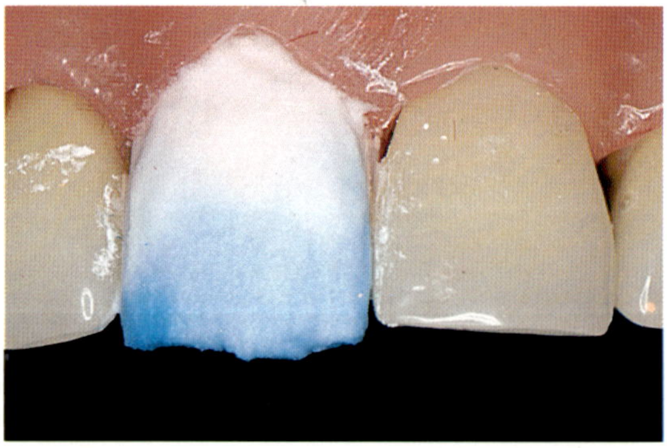

FIG 9–5

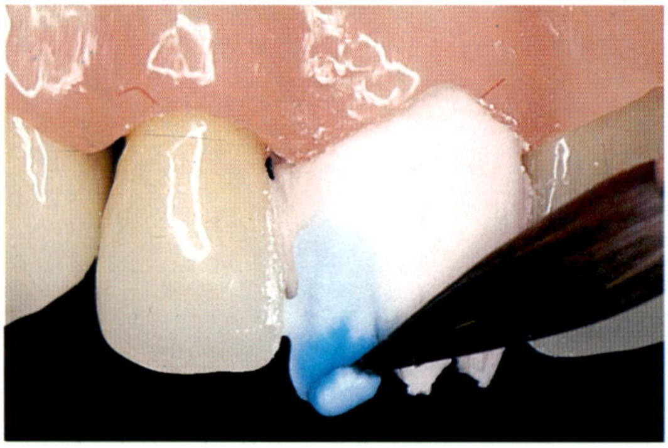

FIG 9–6

All lingual convexities are reduced to the level of the lingual fossa with the curved edge of the grooving blade. The lingual fossa itself is only very superficially scraped. The occlusion is restored in Figure 9–7 with enamel porcelain over the lingual marginal ridges and the cingulum tip.

The translucent powder is mixed with distilled water and applied in continuous progression from the distal to the mesial aspect (Fig 9–8). These incremental additions create a thin coating over the labial incisal and middle thirds and the whole lingual surface. This provides for shrinkage after firing and for additional depth of translucency and refraction. This overlay ideally ranges from 0.2 to 0.3 mm; any thicker coating would produce graying.[1]

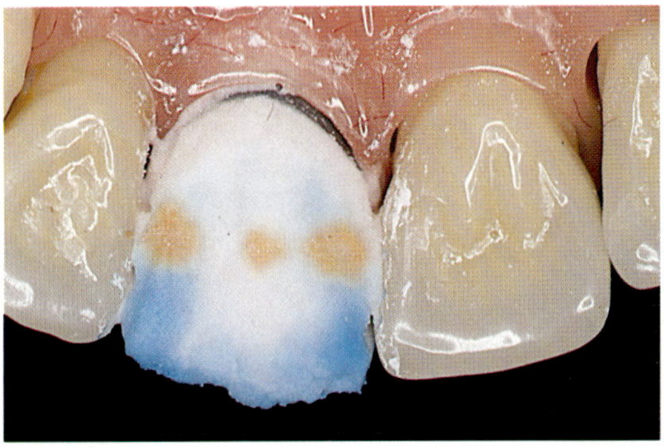

FIG 9–7

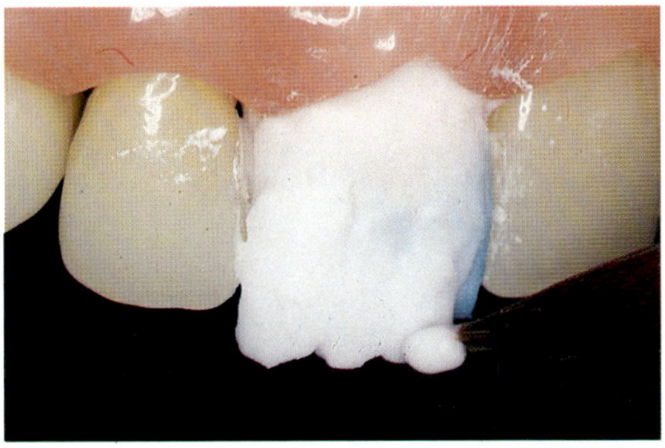

FIG 9–8

Vibration should never be applied at any time during enamel and translucent construction since it could distort the buildup and compromise the sharp boundaries between all three layers. Delicately resurface the labial aspect with the carving blade (Fig 9–9)

Emphasize any depressions with the tip of the brush. Increase the proximal contacts with enamel and translucent porcelain to compensate for shrinkage after firing (Fig 9–10).

Polish the final contours with the large soft-hair brush with no pressure (Figs 9–11 and 9–12).

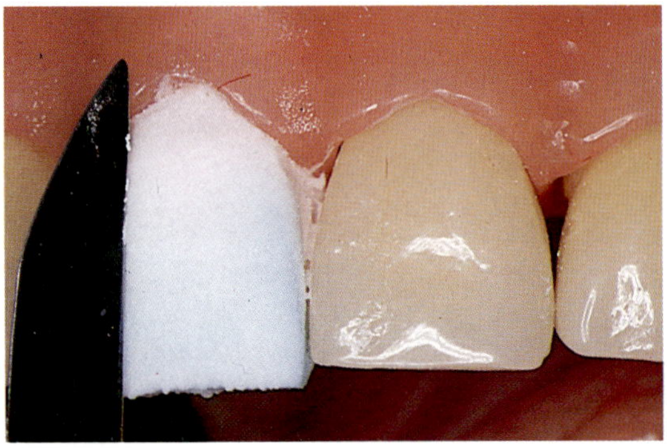

FIG 9–9

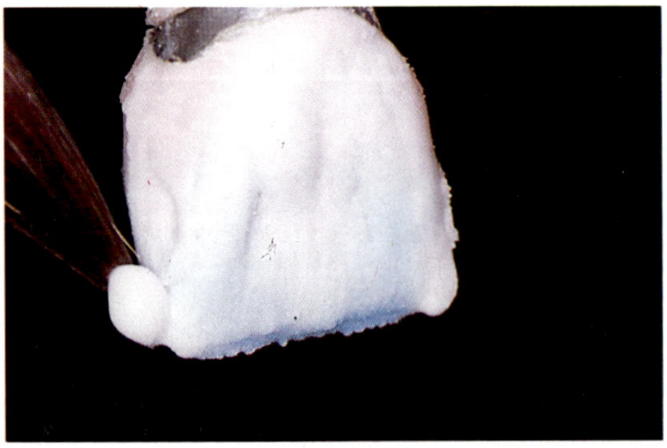

FIG 9–10

Apply, very carefully, two separate ultrasonic vibrations of 1 second each, and absorb any excess water with tissue paper. Distilled water should still comprise 30% to 40% of the weight of body construction. One firing only is indicated prior to glazing.

Finishing is accomplished with diamond and silicon carbide (Carborundum) stones in either sweeping motions or fine, light strokes. The crown must be regularly soaked in water to prevent thermal shock.[2] It would be more convenient to only reemphasize existing surface characteristics on the bisque porcelain rather than recreate them. However, despite the precision of the porcelain construction in the unfired stage, many details will have to be recreated after shrinkage so that they match the adjacent central incisor and impart the same light reflection features. General outlines, including developmental lobes, should already be maintained during the first firing before any finishing is begun.

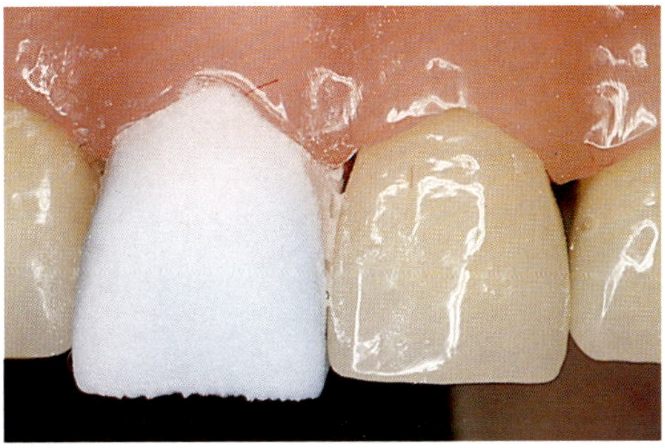

FIG 9–11

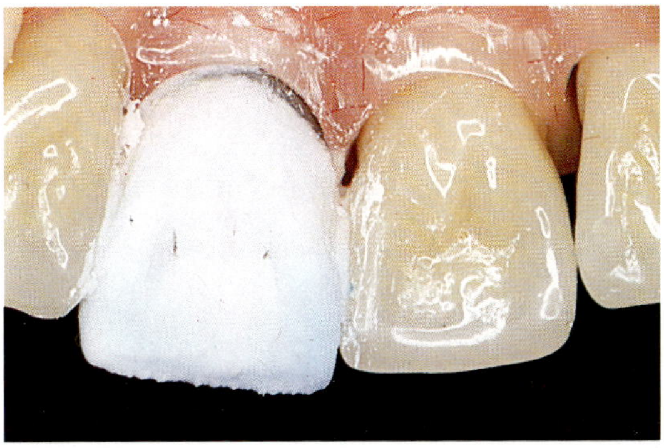

FIG 9–12

The proximal contact areas are adjusted in intensity and size (Fig 9–13). Accurate positioning of the transition line angles produce the desired labial surface width (Fig 9–14). Specific surface reflections are further outlined by emphasizing the triple labial convexity (Fig 9–15). Lobes and depressions are

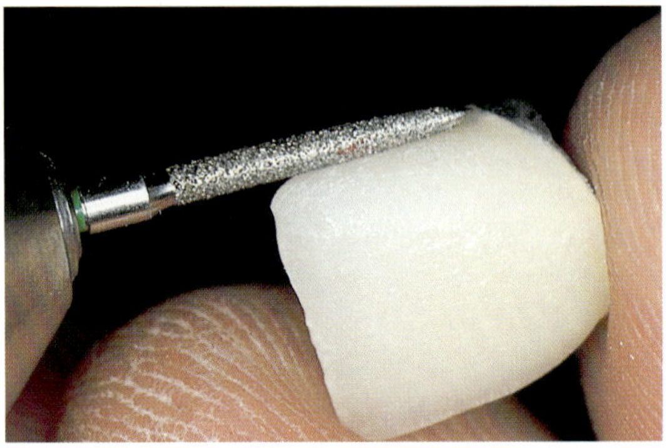

FIG 9–13

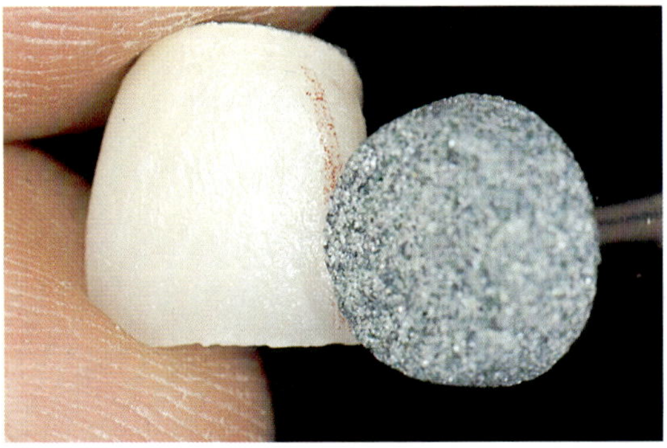

FIG 9–14

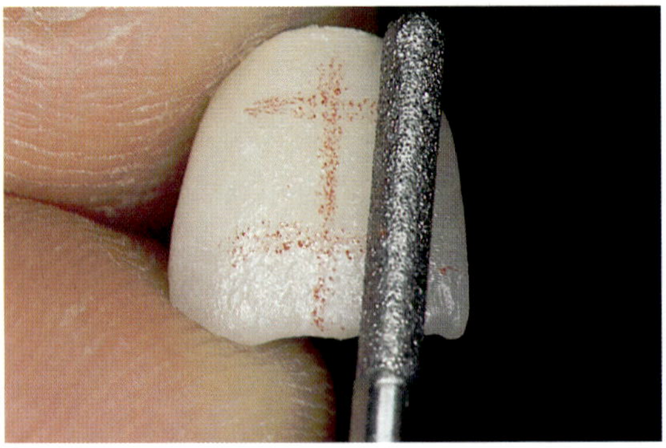

FIG 9–15

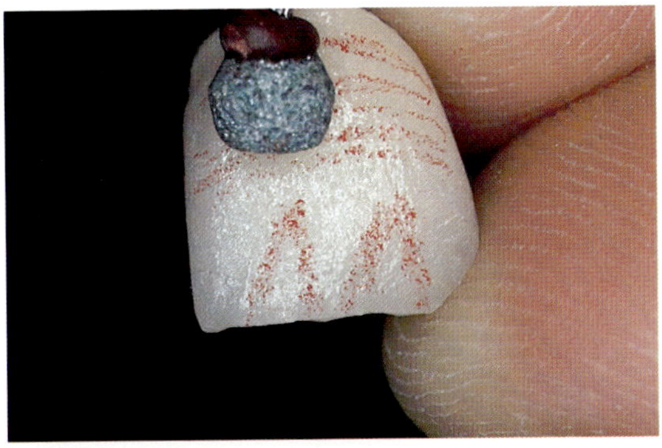

FIG 9–16

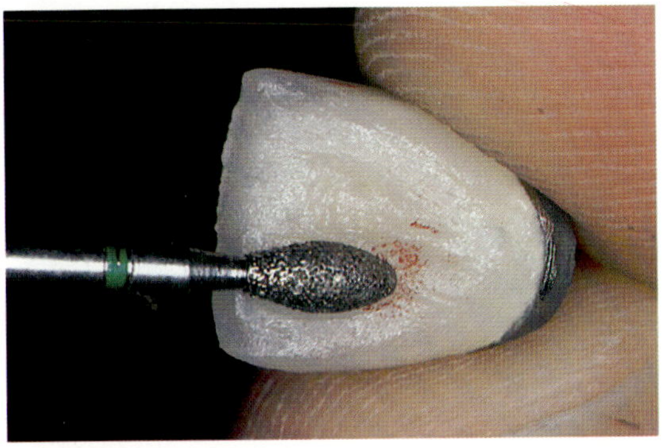

FIG 9–17

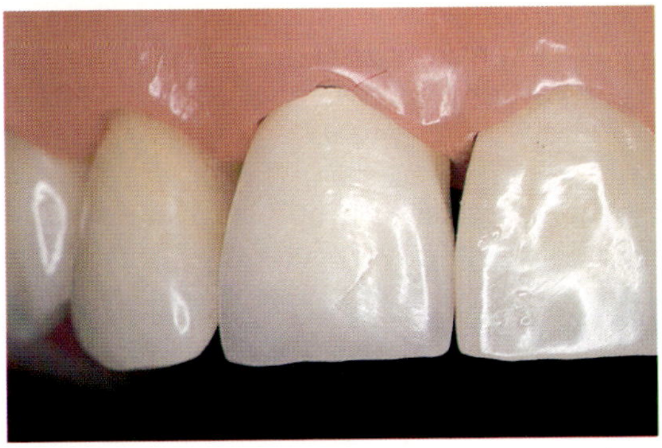

FIG 9–18

also accentuated according to the pattern of the adjacent central incisor (Fig 9–16). Surface perikymatas may also be reproduced when indicated. Adjust the lingual aspect in centric occlusion and in protrusion (Fig 9–17).

Smooth the most prominent ridges with Shofu rubber wheels. Thoroughly clean the crown in ultrasonic solution prior to glazing. Do not apply any surface colorants. Note the high value and reflectivity of the opaque at the cervical margin of the finished crown after glazing in Figure 9–18.

REFERENCES

1. Yamamoto M: *Metal Ceramics*. Chicago, Quintessence Publishing Co, 1985.
2. McLean JW: *The Science and Art of Dental Ceramics*. Chicago, Quintessence Publishing Co, Vol 2, 1980.

Chapter 10

Maxillary Three-Unit Bridge: Three-Powder Construction

All anatomical contours are built to normal dimensions into occlusion except for the incisal edges, which are oversized by 1 mm and the cervical convexities, which are emphasized to compensate for shrinkage. (Refer to Chapter 6 for complete details of the dentin construction.) The amount of labial reduction is determined by the shade prescription. In this exercise (Fig 10–1), it involves the incisal one third of the central incisor and the canine and the labial half of the lateral incisor. Reduce the central incisor first. Bevel the incisal third with the carving blade so that the dentin background is feathered incisally. Cut two labial grooves to develop the three-fingered extension of a mamelon effect. The interproximal reduction is completed last. The proximal contacts must not be broken unless intense effect is desired. The lateral incisor reduction involves the labial half since its enamel coverage is typically greater than on the central incisor. The proximal contact reduction follows the same technique for each unit.

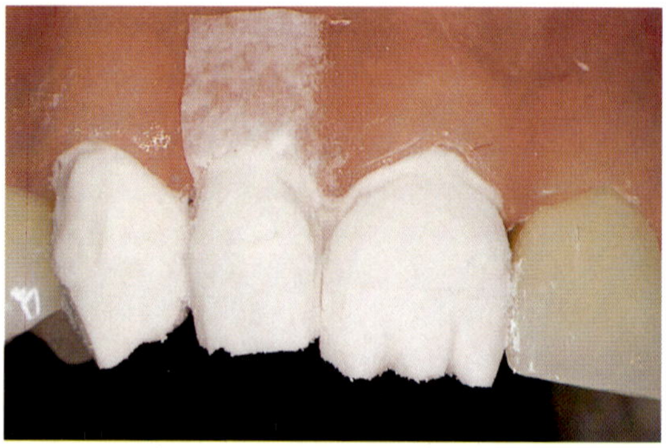

FIG 10–1

The canine reduction involves the incisal third, sometimes less when its saturation needs to be intensified and its translucency decreased in relation to the incisors.

All of these reductions are planned to minimize sharp enamel contrast in the incisal edge and over the proximal contacts and so that the labial dentinoenamel blend line is not demarcated. It is only emphasized on this view for better visualization.

The lingual reductions (Fig 10–2) are made on the lingual ridges and the cingula down to the level of the lingual fossae, which are, in turn, slightly scraped.

Mix enamel powder with distilled water, and restore successively each unit back to full contour (Fig 10–3). The incisal edges are oversized by 1 mm, and

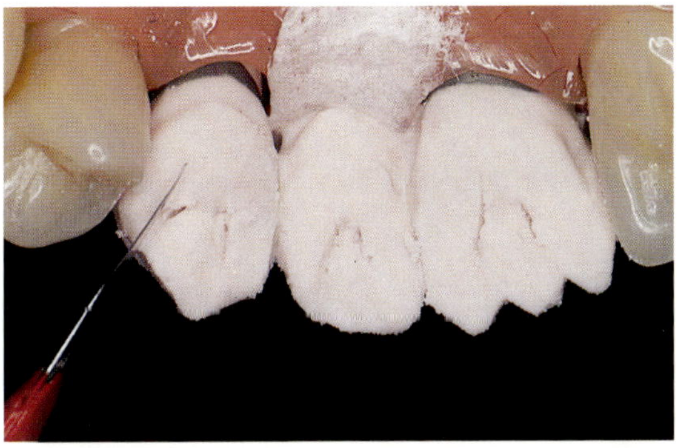

FIG 10–2

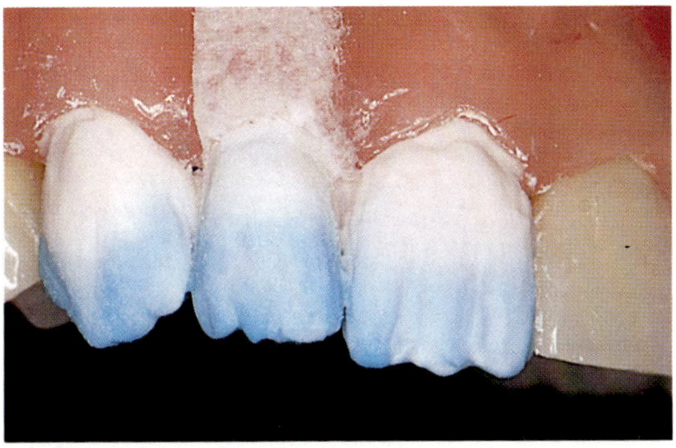

FIG 10–3

the labial lobes are slightly accentuated to compensate for shrinkage. When occlusal clearance is sufficient, it is possible to increase the depth of translucency of the lingual aspect by applying the enamel over the lingual ridges and the cingulum but keeping it slightly out of occlusion (Fig 10–4), so that the thickness of the translucent overlay can be increased. Mix translucent powder with distilled water, and coat the labial two thirds of each unit (Fig 10–5). This provides for shrinkage compensation, additional depth of translucency, and internal refraction. The carving blade is used interproximally to emphasize individuality (Fig 10–6). The incisal pin of the articulator is elevated by 1 mm, and the occlusion

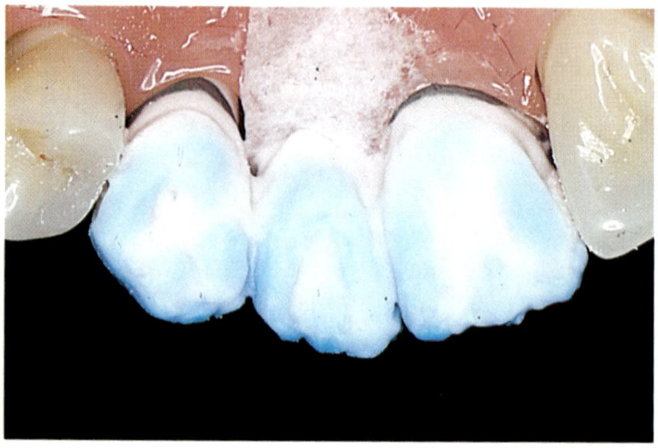

FIG 10–4

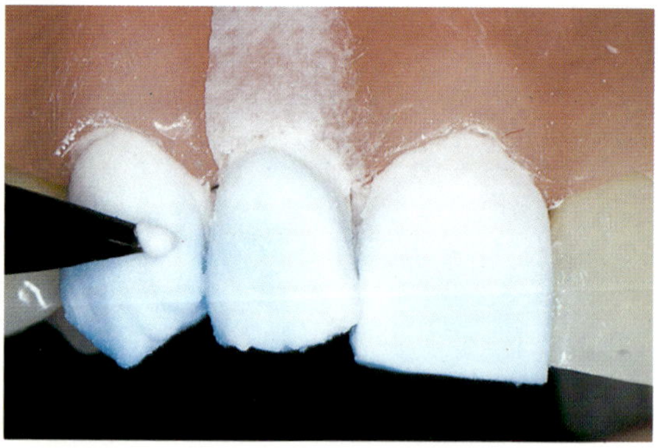

FIG 10–5

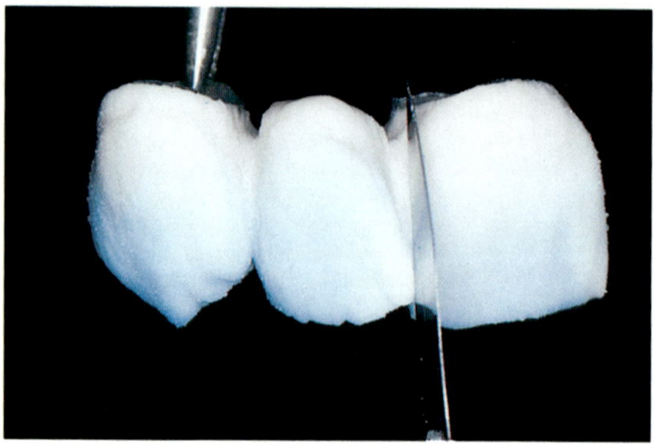

FIG 10–6

is restored with translucent porcelain (Fig 10–7). The protrusive pathways are checked very delicately to avoid buildup fracture. Proximal contacts are enlarged with enamel overlaid with translucent (Fig 10–8). Apply two separate ultrasonic vibrations of 1 second each, and carefully absorb any excess moisture.

After firing (Fig 10–9), enamel distribution is subtle. Labial and lingual additions, where needed, are made with a mixture of equal parts of dentin and translucent over the developmental ridges, and translucent only for superficial alterations (Fig 10–10). After the second firing, recreate and highlight surface

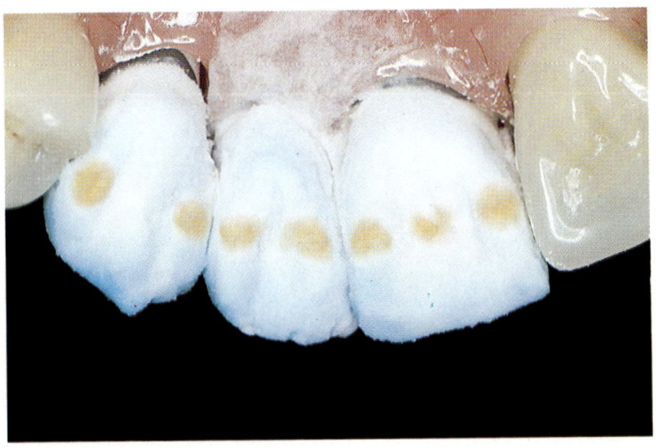

FIG 10–7

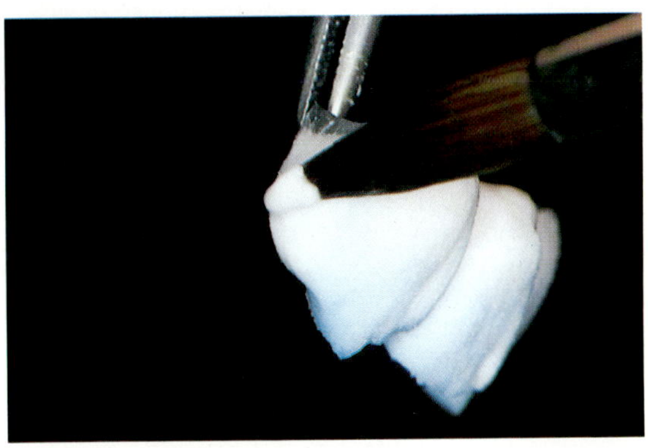

FIG 10–8

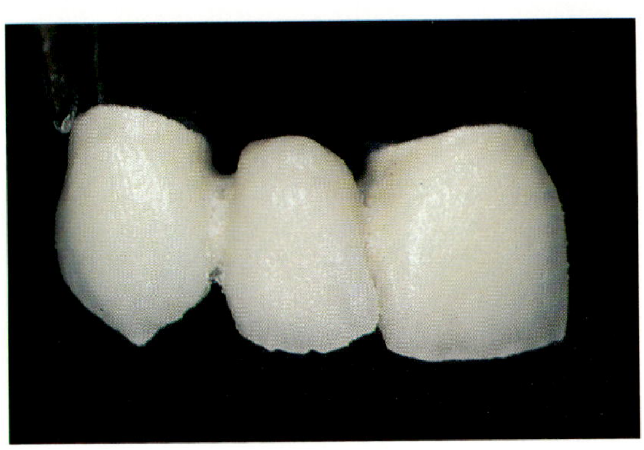

FIG 10–9

characteristics (see Chapter 9). Reemphasize individuality with a diamond disc (Fig 10–11). Smooth the most prominent ridges with Shofu rubber wheels, and thoroughly clean the crown in ultrasonic solution. Only dark brown surface stain mixed with 1 part of stain liquid to 10 parts of distilled water is applied with a fine staining sable brush in the embrasures to accentuate depth and individuality.

Note the final result after glazing in Figure 10–12.

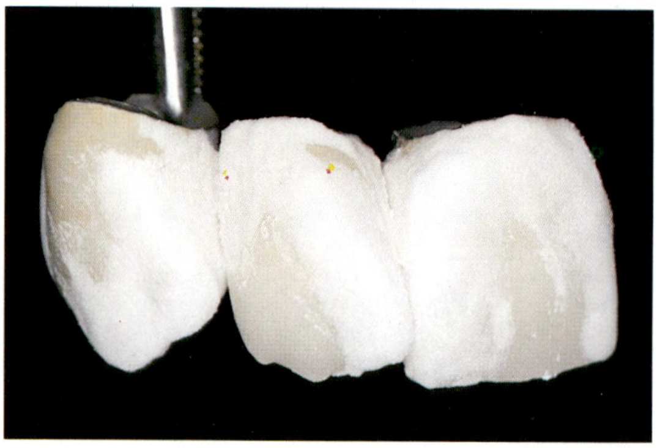

FIG 10–10

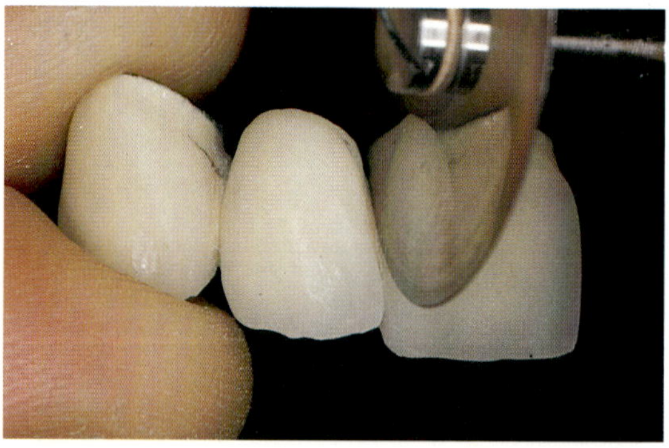

FIG 10–11

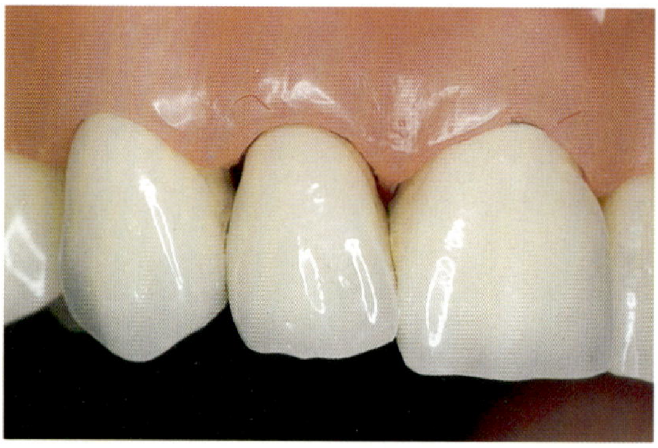

FIG 10–12

Chapter 11

Maxillary First Molar: Three-Powder Construction

All anatomical contours are built to normal dimensions and in maximum intercuspation as described in Chapter 5.

The cervical region is slightly oversized to compensate for shrinkage since it will neither be reduced nor overlaid.

The axial reductions are performed with the carving blade. The labial reduction extends slightly below the incisal third level. The beveling creates a gradual fading of the dentin background but may vary according to the shade prescription. Each axial cusp plane is carved separately so that a dentin core is preserved inside each cusp (Fig 11–1).

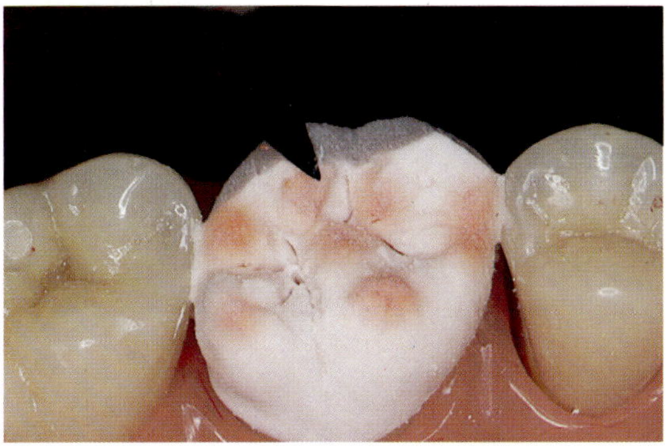

FIG 11–1

The angulation of the carving blade must respect each axial cuspal plane (Figs 11–2 and 11–3). The occlusal reductions are performed with the curved edge of the grooving blade. The reduction maintains the outline of the cusp and developmental grooves. The inner inclines of every cusp are flattened for complete elimination of the triangular ridges (Fig 11–4). These will be formed with

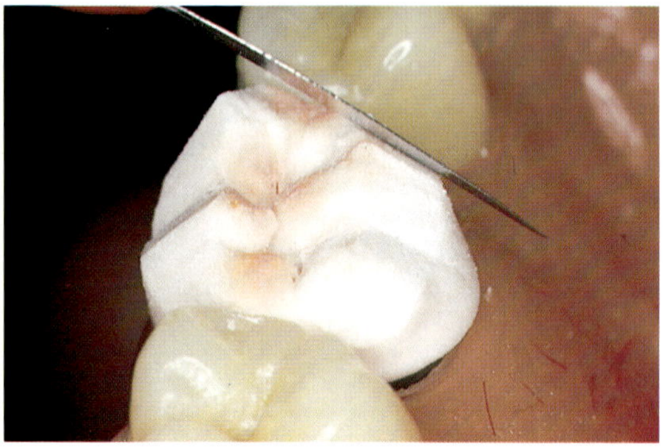

FIG 11–2

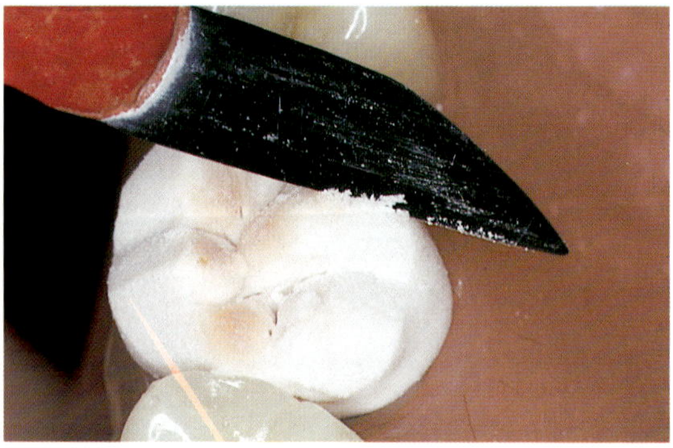

FIG 11–3

enamel and translucent porcelain only. The marginal ridges are carved back without breaking proximal contacts to avoid sharp color demarcation with the rest of the construction. The completed reduction allocates the necessary space for enamel porcelain. It preserves cusp and fossa outlines but eliminates internal convexities (Fig 11–5). Residual dentin thickness ranges from 0.7 to 1 mm.

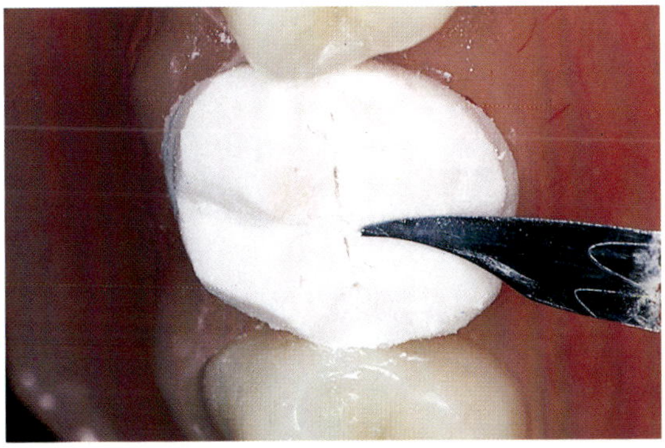

FIG 11–4

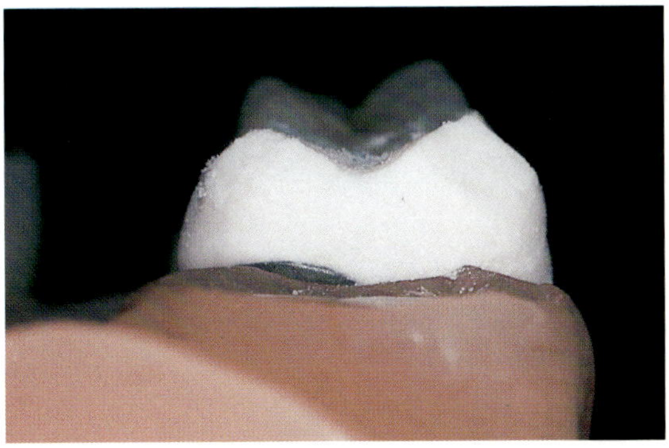

FIG 11–5

Enamel powder is mixed with distilled water and must be applied in increments (Fig 11–6).

Labial contours are restored back to normal dimensions with enamel porcelain from the cusp tip down.

Lingual contours are restored back to occlusion in enamel porcelain. Press the cusp tips with the buildup brush to a different position if necessary (Fig 11–7).

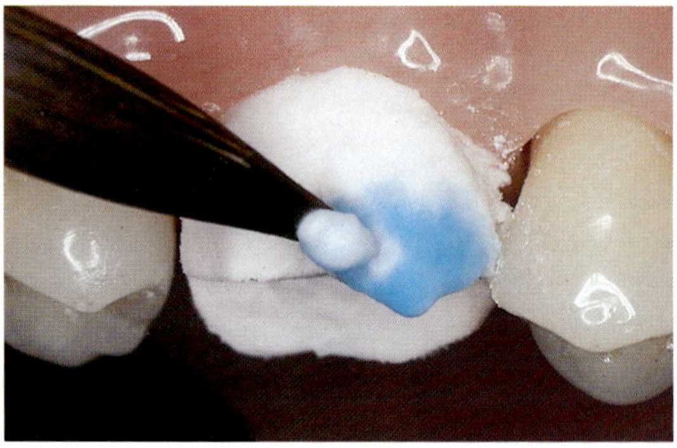

FIG 11–6

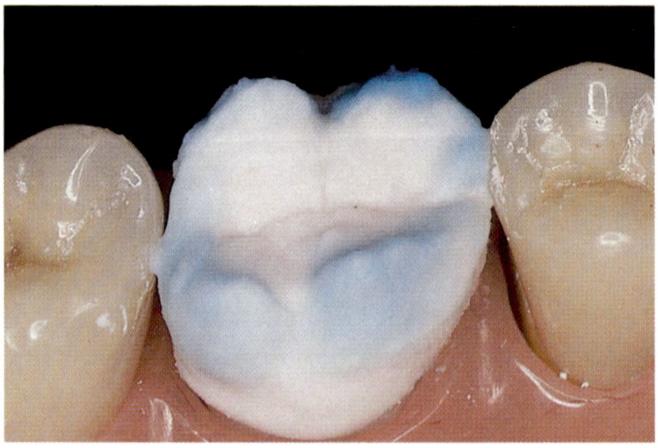

FIG 11–7

The marginal and triangular ridges are formed slightly out of occlusion to provide additional space for the translucent powder. Check the occlusion. Only the centric cusps are in contact (Fig 11–8). Elevate the articulator pin by 1 mm. Mix translucent powder in distilled water, and apply it in increments.

Overlay the labial aspect with a thin coat, covering the incisal and the middle third (Fig 11–9). It is oversized incisally by 1 mm on each cusp.

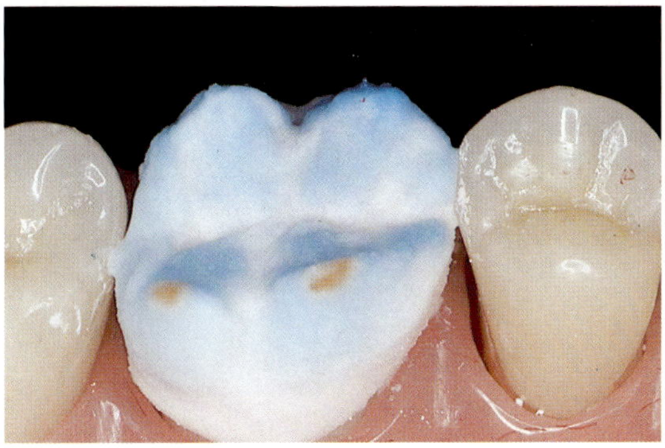

FIG 11–8

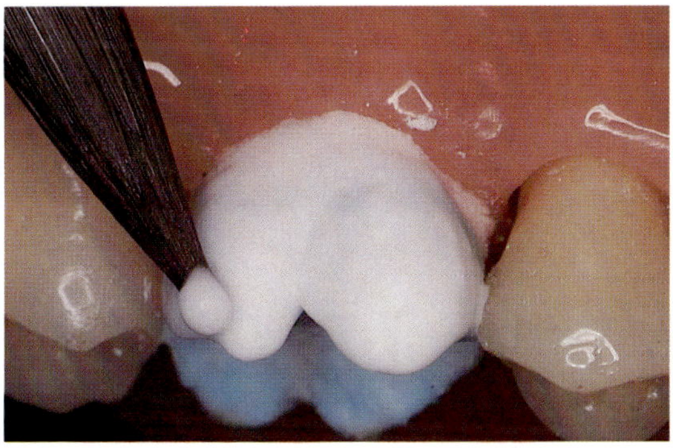

FIG 11–9

Overlay the lingual aspect and build the lingual cusps into the elevated new occlusion (Fig 11–10).

Restore the triangular ridges to the new occlusion by pulling the translucent porcelain beads from the cusp tip down to the fossa (Fig 11–11).

Progress by continuity to the marginal ridges and to the labial triangular ridges with small lobulated additions. Check the occlusion for major interferences; be careful not to detach or break the buildup from its foundation during lateral excursions.

Finish and polish all axial contours with the large soft-hair brush.

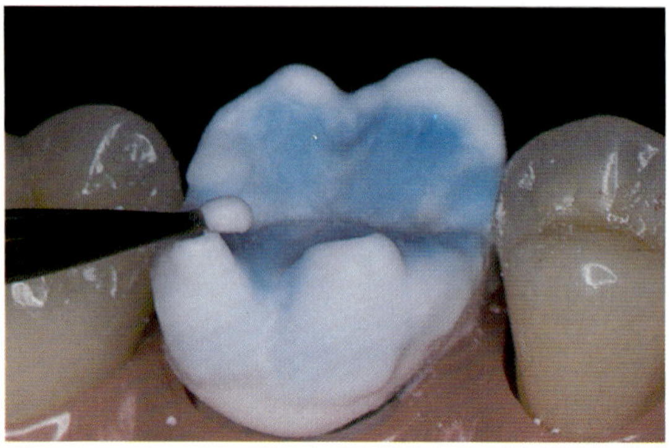

FIG 11–10

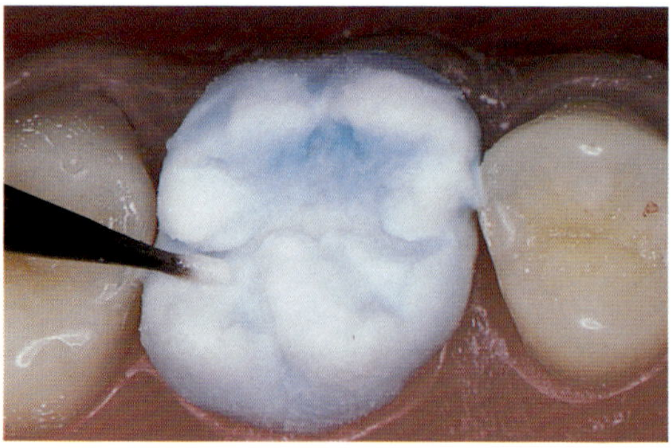

FIG 11–11

Refine the developmental and supplemental grooves with the tip of the fine sable-hair brush and accessorily the grooving blade.

Lightly polish the occlusal surface with the large soft-hair brush. Apply two separate ultrasonic vibrations of 1 second each, and absorb the excess moisture with tissue paper. Deepen the occlusal pits with the point of the grooving blade (Fig 11–12). This will ensure that each cusp may shrink separately during firing without tearing the grooves apart. Enlarge the proximal contact areas with enamel overlaid with translucent porcelain (Fig 11–13). The precision of the buildup is essential. Mistakes made during construction of the unfired porcelain are

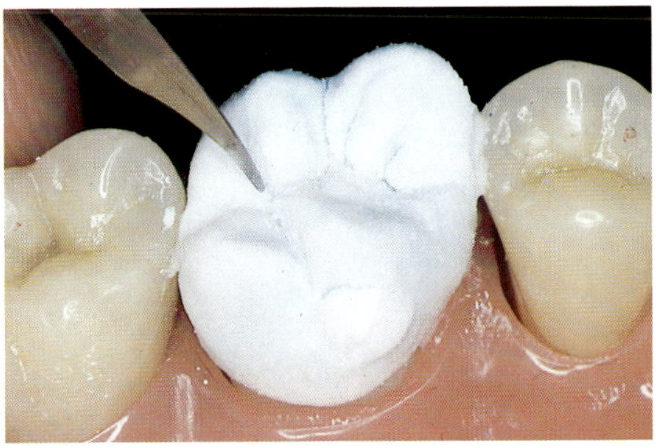

FIG 11–12

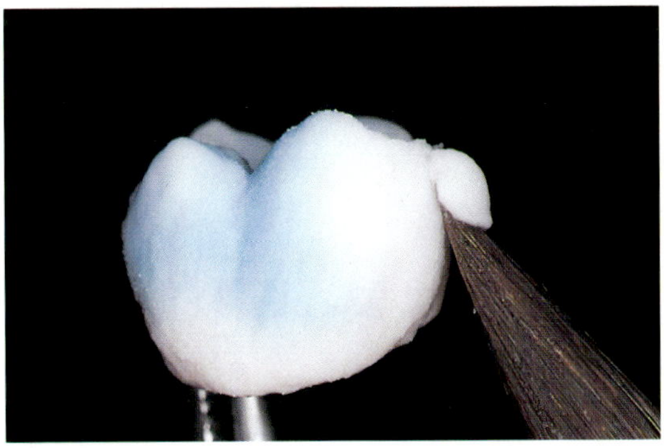

FIG 11–13

irreversible. After first firing, notice the enamel and translucent distribution. The anatomy will need only to be refined, but not recreated (Fig 11–14).

Finishing is accomplished with diamond stones and carbide burs. (See Chapter 14 for more details.) The ridge and groove pattern needs minimum alterations.

Occlusal prematurities are adjusted until harmonious occlusion is created (Fig 11–15). Clean the crown thoroughly in ultrasonic solution. All single units should be completed in one body firing to preserve translucency.

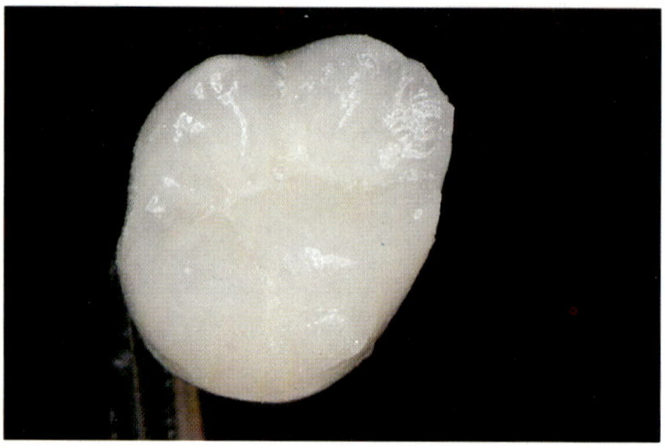

FIG 11–14

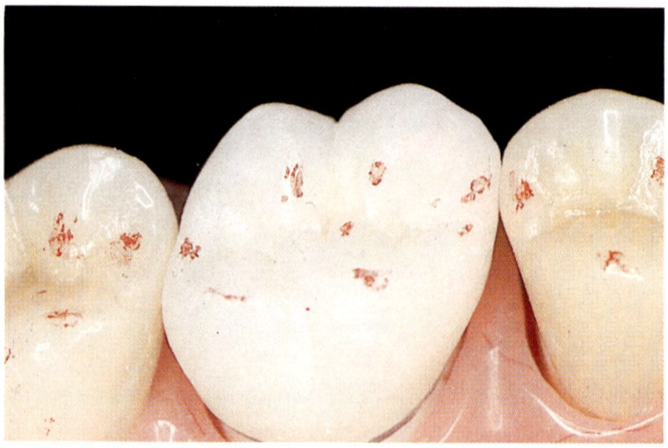

FIG 11–15

Figures 11–16 and 11–17 show the final result after glazing. An equal mix of black with brown surface colorants is applied only in occlusal pits, and dark brown is scattered along the developmental grooves. Figure 11–18 shows the labial view; the translucent and enamel progression over the dentin is gradual, including the proximal areas.

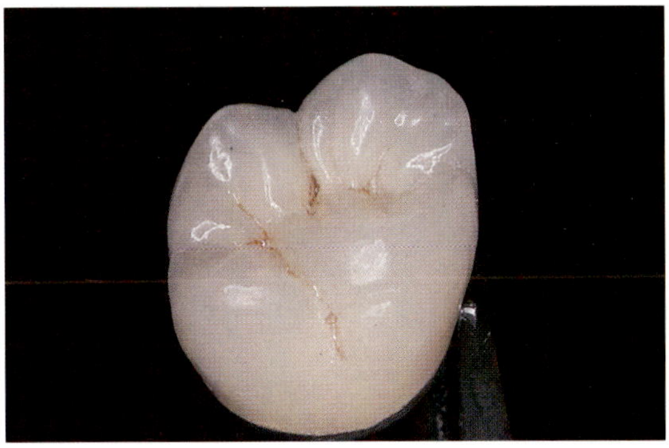

FIG 11–16

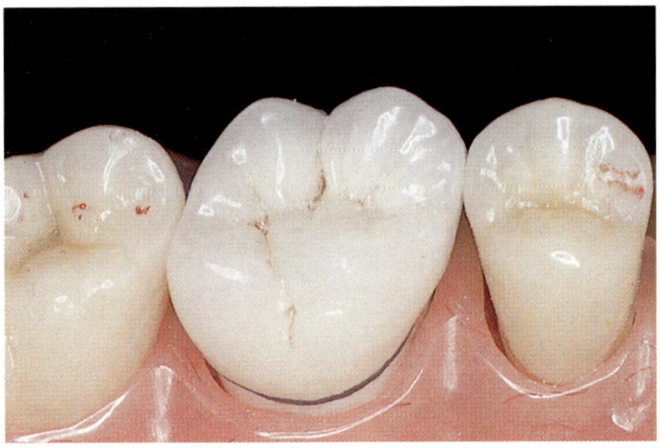

FIG 11–17

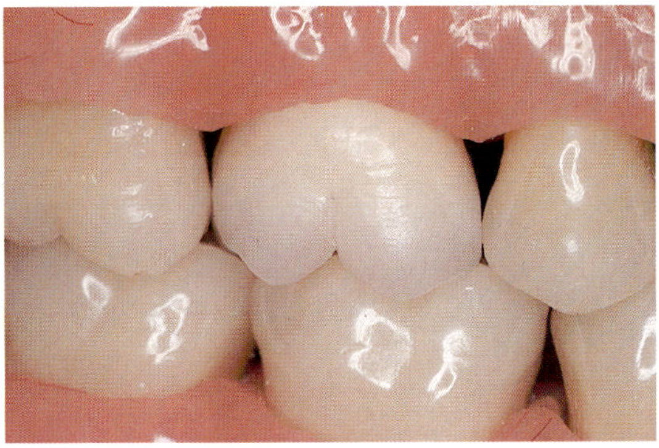

FIG 11–18

Chapter 12

Mandibular Three-Unit Bridge: Three-Powder Construction

All anatomical contours are built in dentin to normal dimensions in maximum intercuspation as described in Chapter 6. The cervical regions are slightly oversized to compensate for shrinkage. To prolong working time, opaque liquid is mixed with distilled water for the dentin construction only in the proportion of 1 to 8.

The axial reductions are made with the carving blade (Fig 12–1).

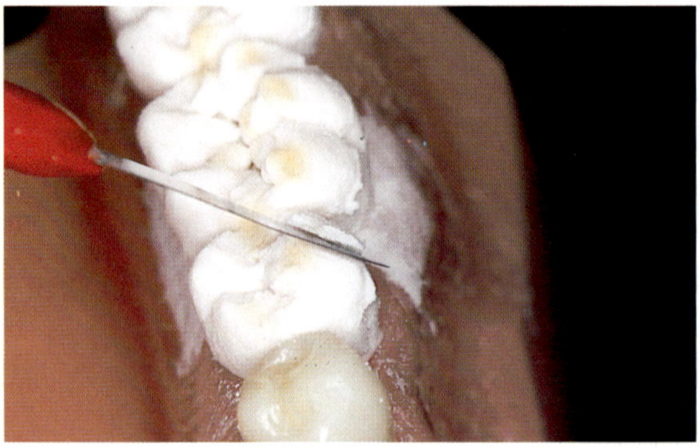

FIG 12–1

The labial reductions extend slightly below the incisal third bevel and vary according to the shade prescription. The beveling creates a gradual fading of the dentin background. Each axial cuspal plane is carved separately to preserve a dentin core inside each cusp (Fig 12–2).

Repeat the same procedure on each lingual cusp.

The occlusal reductions are made with the curved edge of the grooving blade (Fig 12–3). They maintain the outline of the cusp and developmental grooves.

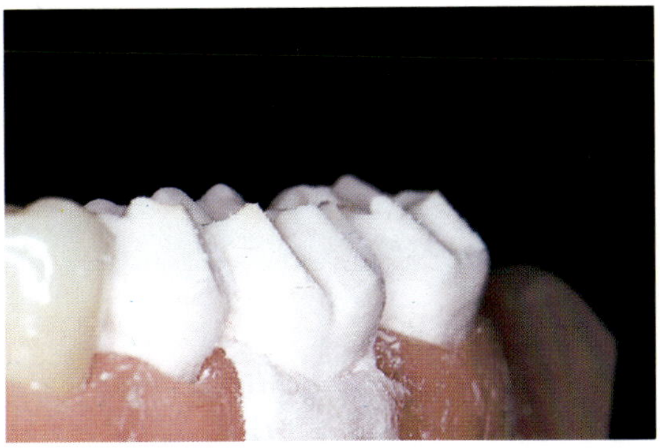

FIG 12–2

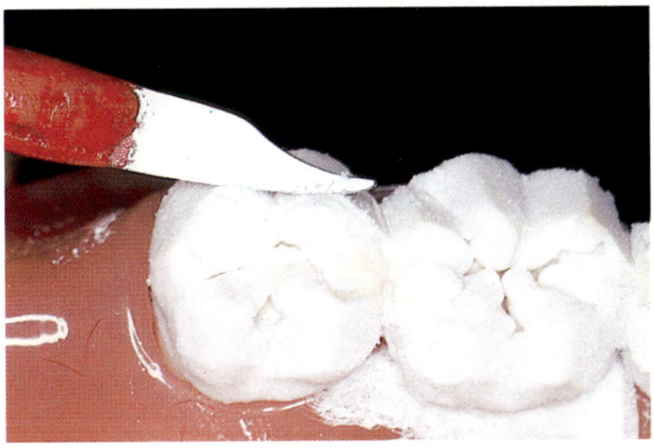

FIG 12–3

The inner inclines of every cusp are flattened for complete elimination of the triangular ridges, which will be formed in enamel and translucent porcelains only (Fig 12–4). The marginal ridges are carved back without breaking proximal contacts. The objectives of the reduction are to preserve dentin color and to allocate sufficient space for enamel porcelain. It maintains cusp and fossa outlines but eliminates internal convexities (Fig 12–5). Residual dentin thickness ranges from 0.7 to 1 mm.

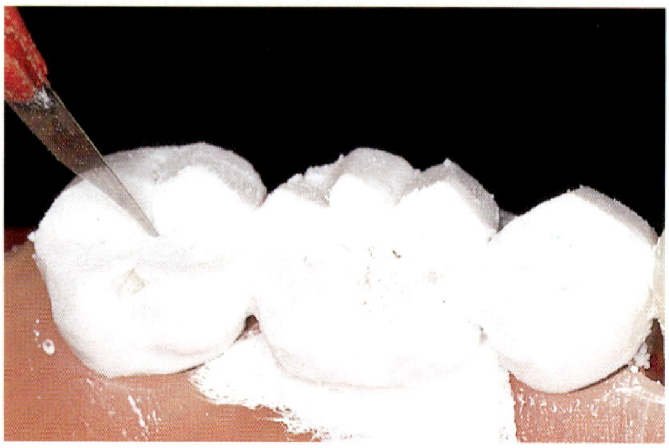

FIG 12–4

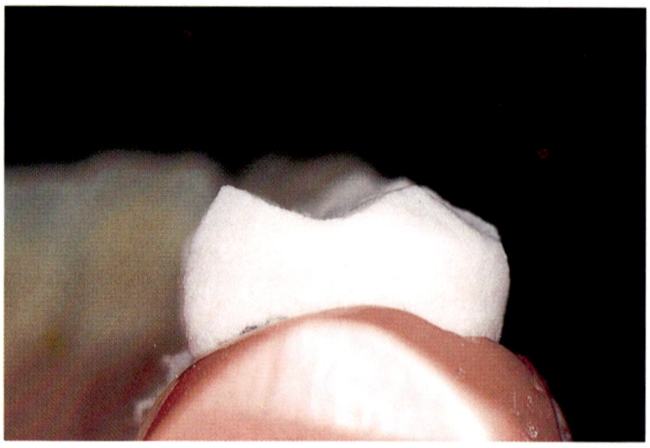

FIG 12–5

Mix enamel powder with distilled water, and apply in increments (Fig 12–6). Restore labial contours back to occlusion with enamel porcelain from each cusp tip down. Feather each lobe addition as it reaches the junction of the incisal and middle third. Press the cusp tip with the buildup brush to a different position if necessary. Build back the lingual contours to normal dimensions with enamel porcelain (Fig 12–7). The marginal and triangular ridges should be formed slightly out of occlusion to provide for additional space for the translucent porcelain and for better depth of translucency. Check the occlusal contacts. Only the centric cusps should be in occlusion at this stage (Fig 12–8).

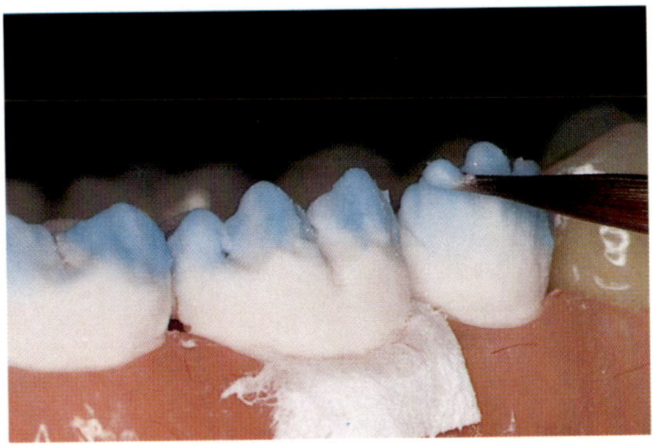

FIG 12–6

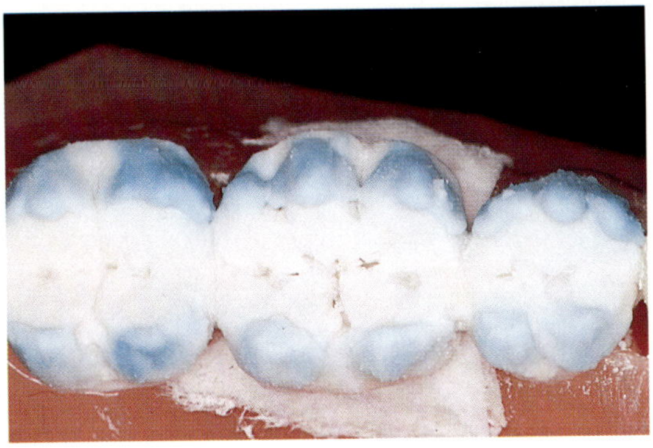

FIG 12–7

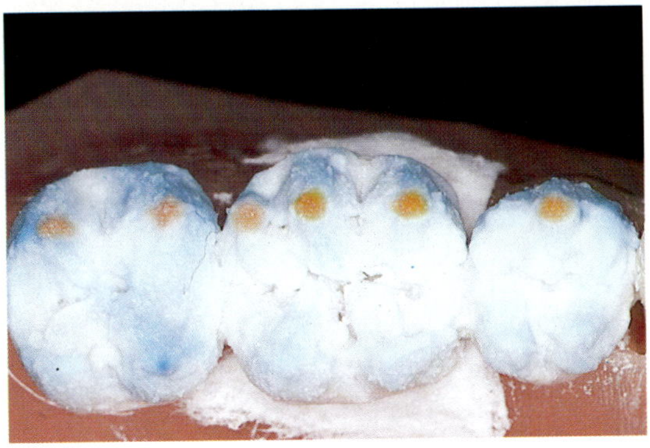

FIG 12–8

Elevate the articulator pin by 1 mm.

Mix translucent powder with distilled water only, and apply it in increments (Fig 12–9). Successively overlay each labial cusp with lobulated additions. Restore them into occlusion from the tip down. Extend the coating over the incisal and middle third (Fig 12–10).

Overlay the lingual cusp and oversize them in length by 1 mm. Restore the triangular ridges by pulling the translucent porcelain beads from cusp tip to fossa (Fig 12–11). The buildup may saturate with excessive water, and surface

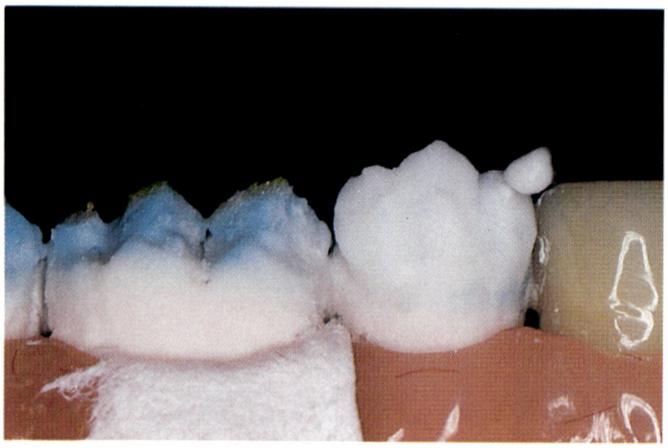

FIG 12–9

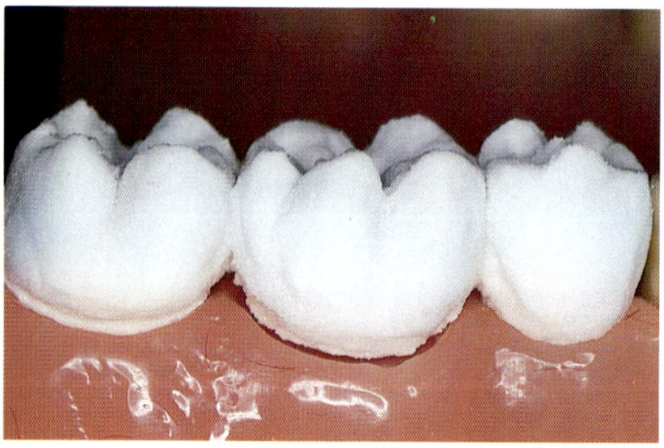

FIG 12–10

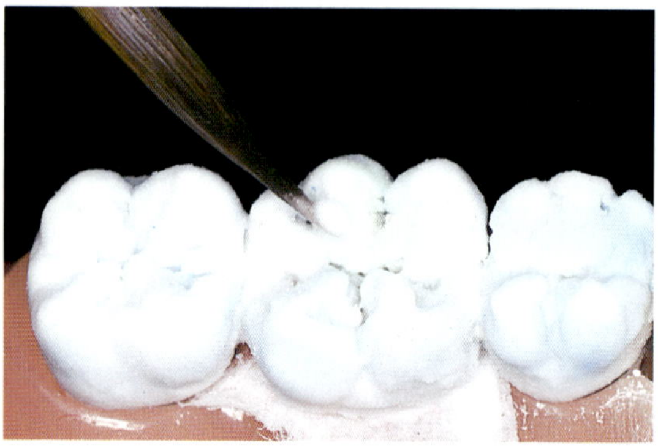

FIG 12–11

details may be blurred. Proceed from one unit to the next back and forth to allow for some evaporation to take place. Never vibrate during the construction. The marginal ridge additions are very delicate because they must restore individuality between each unit. Check the occlusion for major interferences. Be careful not to detach or break the buildup from its base.

Finish and polish the axial contours with the large soft-hair brush. Refine the developmental and supplemental grooves with the tip of the fine sable-hair brush (Fig 12–12). Lightly polish the occlusal surfaces with the large soft-hair brush. Apply two separate ultrasonic vibrations of 1 second each, and absorb the excess moisture with tissue paper. Deepen the occlusal pits with the point of the grooving blade so that each cusp shrinks separately during firing without tearing the grooves apart. Enlarge the proximal contacts with enamel covered with translucent porcelain. Refine the underside of the pontic into a modified ridge lap design. The precision and the buildup is essential. Mistakes made during construction of the unfired porcelain are irreversible (Fig 12–13).

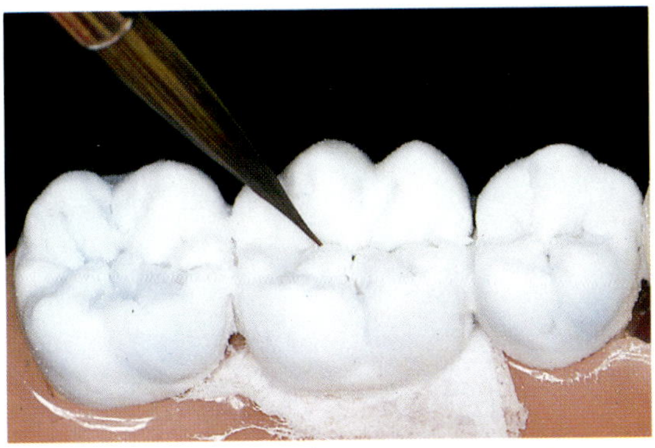

FIG 12–12

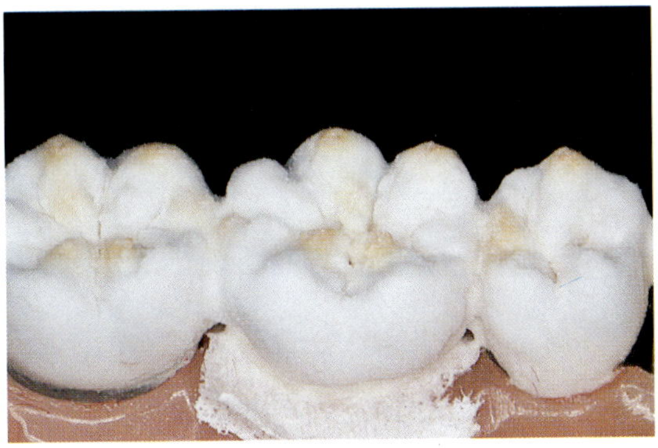

FIG 12–13

The bridge is predried over the firing tray for 9 minutes (Fig 12–14). After first firing, shrinkage is significant, but outlines and color distribution are preserved (Fig 12–15).

Additions are made with dentin and translucent mixed in equal parts over the cervical third, enamel and translucent mixed in equal parts over the middle third, and translucent over the incisal third and the occlusal surface. Any missing occlusal contact is restored in this phase (Fig 12–16).

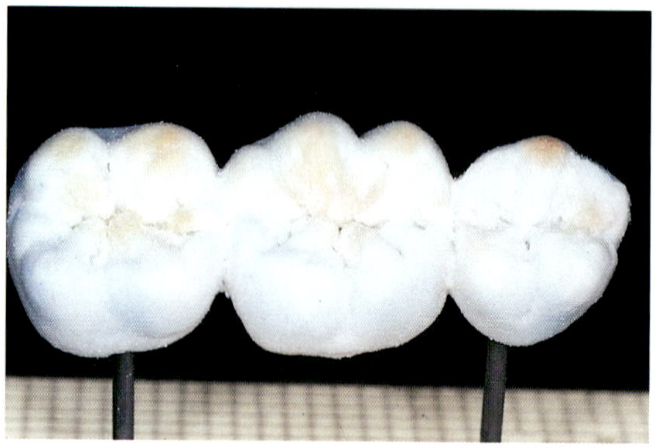

FIG 12–14

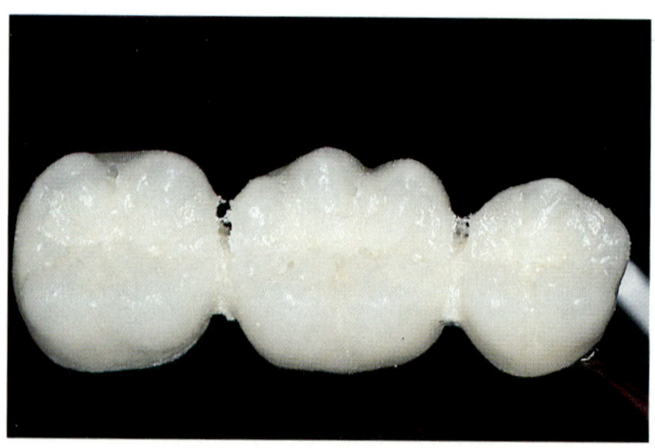

FIG 12–15

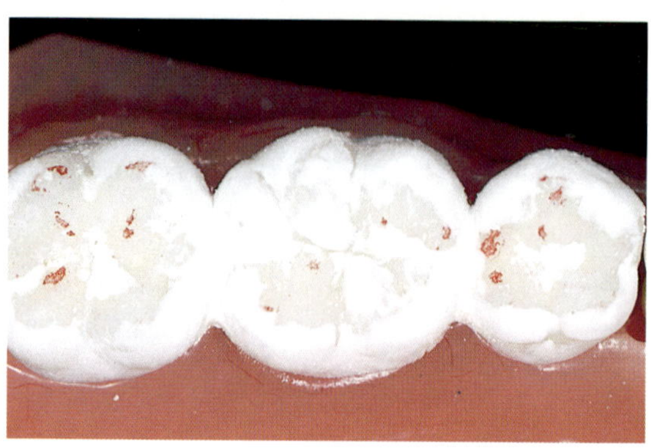

FIG 12–16

The second firing is performed at a reduced temperature (−15°C) and higher firing rate (10°C).

After firing, the anatomy needs to be refined but not recreated. Finishing is accomplished with diamond stones and carbide burs (see Chapter 14). The ridge and groove pattern needs only minimum alterations. Occlusal prematurities are adjusted until harmonious occlusion is achieved (Fig 12–17). Clean the bridge thoroughly in ultrasonic solution. Figure 12–18 shows the completed bridge after glazing. An equal mix of black and brown surface colorant was applied in the occlusal pits, and dark brown was scattered along the developmental grooves.

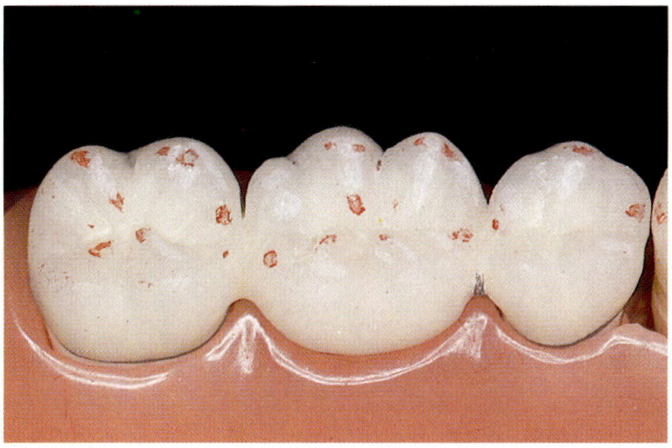

FIG 12–17

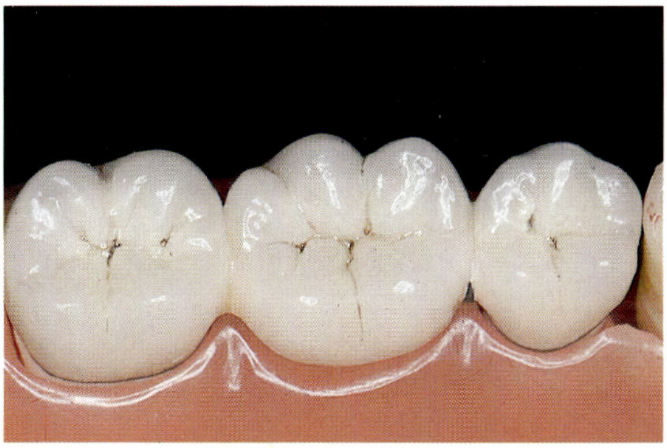

FIG 12–18

Chapter 13

Internal Shading

In porcelain construction, color should be elaborated in depth since dentin is the primary source of natural tooth color. This arrangement takes full advantage of the softening and filtering effect of enamel. The main difficulty is that shade correction of the final crown may not be possible if its value is too low. Also, predicting internal color after firing requires a great deal of experience; this may frustrate the beginner and result in a stronger reliance on external staining.

External shading may be associated with obvious, sometimes excessive, characterizations that replicate decalcifications or discolorations (Fig 13–1), but from

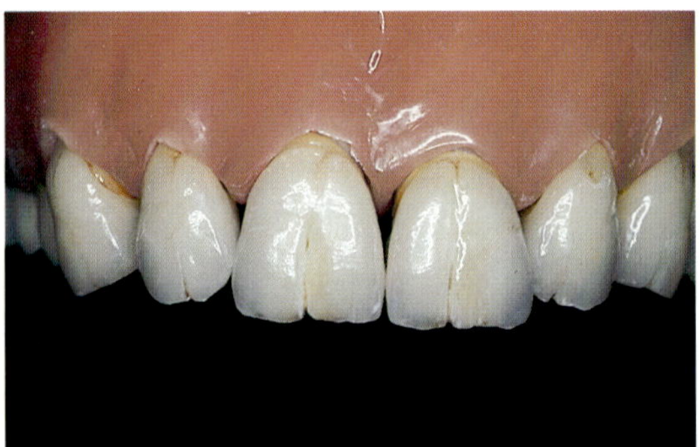

FIG 13–1

a cultural standpoint, many patients may object to such realism unless the crowns match their natural adjacent teeth. Internal shading is generally quite subtle, and it is intended to transmit internal color through enamel and enhance form perception by the observer. Translucency and internal refraction always remain essential considerations during porcelain construction and firing. No matter how complex the layering pattern is, there should be a distinct boundary between each layer (Fig 13–2).[1, 2]

OPAQUE MODIFICATIONS

Opaque modifications are indicated where porcelain thickness is minimum, when value needs to be reduced through strong internal effects, or when depth and saturation must be emphasized. The deeper the modifications, the less prominent its effect on the overall color.[3] Therefore, under ideal dentin and enamel thickness, opaque modification is significant only at the cervical edge and in the embrasures for depth and individuality. Cervical saturation and depth can be accentuated with orange mixed with brown or with orange modifiers or with an opaque of a darker shade. Depth perception is reinforced with orange modifiers over the fossa area and violet modifier mixed with white over the cusp elevations.

CERVICAL SHADING

Cervical shading is dictated by the shade prescription, which assesses the cervical saturation of the tooth to match that of the shade tab. It is replicated with a high chroma porcelain (cervical or gingival porcelain) mixed in proportions ranging from 1 to 7 to 10 parts of regular dentin according to the desired effect. The prescription should also incorporate any possible orange tonality. Most shade guides are confined only to yellow hues,[4–6] whereas up to 50% of extracted teeth studied visually or under spectophotometry[7–10] extend into the yellow-red

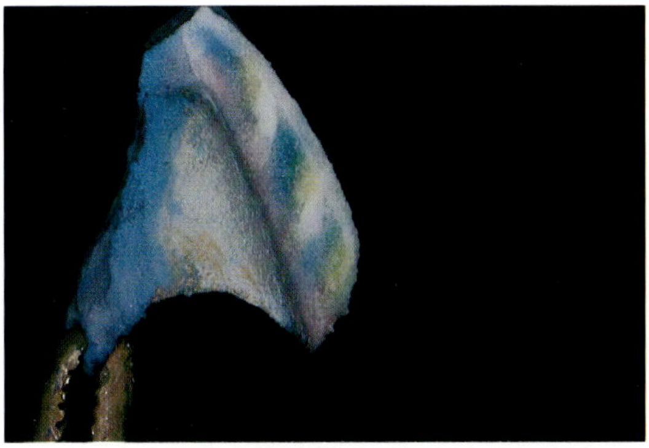

FIG 13–2

(orange) color space. Even though these findings are extrapolated from extracted teeth to natural teeth in vivo, they are substantiated by daily clinical practice. The orange component, when detected, is most conspicuous in the cervical region, where enamel is thinnest, and is reproduced with orange powder mixed in proportions ranging from 1 to 5 parts to 10 parts of regular dentin according to the desired effect. The saturation and the extent of the cervical hue can increase with age, because, in many instances, calcification is most evident at the cervix before progressing incisally.[2] It is also influenced by any slight root exposure, which projects a shadow that is interpreted as additional saturation. The opposite is also quite often encountered where the cervix appears to be the least saturated part of the whole tooth, especially in the absence of gingival recession, and appears very distinctly during tooth preparation as a brighter band (Fig 13–3).[11] Regular opaque modification will not be compatible with this arrangement, which requires higher cervical value. This, in turn, would not effectively mask the gray oxidation metal line. It is solved with either a shoulder porcelain design, eliminating metal and opaque from the margin, or a coat of 70% opacious dentin mixed with 30% dentin applied after opaque firing.

Adjustment of cervical chroma, especially when contrasting with opalescent enamel, creates pleasing, dynamic shade patterns, provided natural translucency is maintained at the cervix (Fig 13–4). Translucency is directly affected by metal

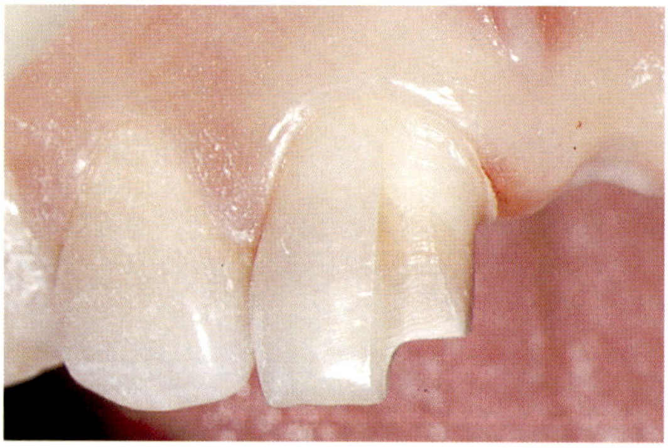

FIG 13–3

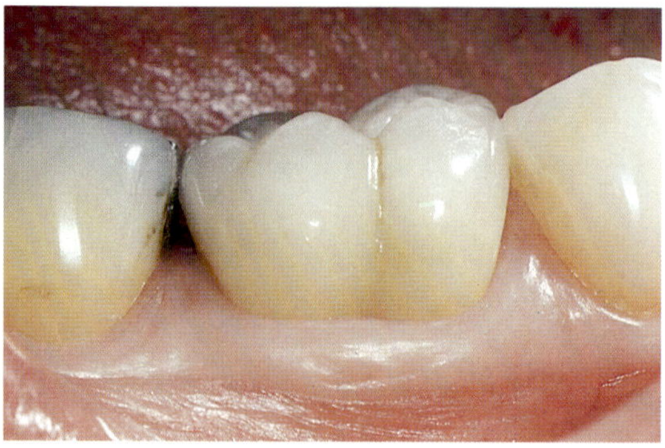

FIG 13–4

porcelain design. When properly constructed, shoulder porcelain margins yield the best results[12] since they avoid metal and opaque influence at the finish line and shadowing over the root. Excellent but slightly inferior performances result from the gold-ceramic design with a hairline metal collar.[2]

The next best compromise is modified or darker opaque or opacious dentin over unmodified opaque, with a hairline metal collar. In all of these designs, very light applications of surface colorants just prior to glazing may be applied to reach the precise final shade. Unmodified opaque with cervical porcelain corrected only with surface colorants at the staining and glazing stage may be acceptable, but definitely compromise cervical translucency and may never mask opaque brightness adequately. This is evident in Figure 13–5 in the molar on the left side, compared with a modified opaque design overlaid with cervical porcelain mixed with orange, shown on the right.

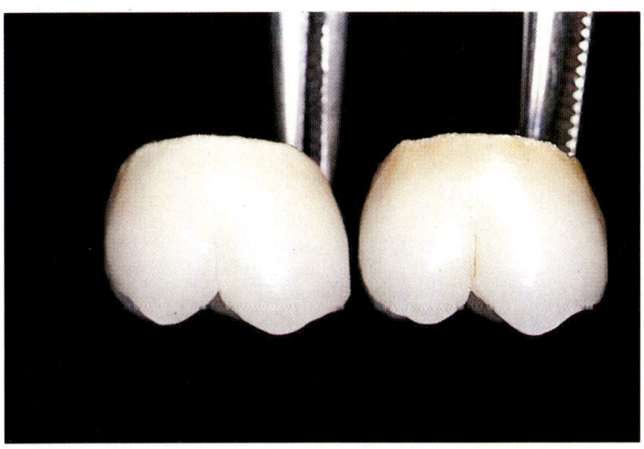

FIG 13–5

BODY SHADING

Optimum shade is best achieved under ideal porcelain thickness,[4, 13] which is especially critical for lighter shades.[14] Buildup of full contours is mandatory; it establishes the basic hue and provides for an accurate reference from which precise reduction (cutback) and overlaps are made.

In situations where thickness may be problematic, a preliminary application of a thin coat of opacious dentin[15] neutralizes the opaque layer so that the regular body replicates the shade. It also prevents shadowing and graying in the embrasures. In more compromised instances, colored effects may have to be directly painted over dentin. For example, violet beneath the enamel could mimic opalescence.

Depth and shadowing are simulated next with pure orange or light brown in the embrasure and the occlusal fossa and with an orange-brown combination under the developmental grooves of posterior teeth. The dentin body shading also contributes to enhance labial convexity with interspersion of the lightest possible dentin (A1, B1, etc.), pure or mixed with 10% white. A typical dynamic progression creates a vibrant color effect, as depicted on this bridge retainer over the second premolar against the natural first premolar (Fig 13–6). At the cervical margin, over the first millimeter, A2 is mixed with 2 parts per 10 parts of orange; this lighter tone slightly contrasts with the cervical infrabulge of A3 mixed with 2 parts per 10 parts of orange. The main convexity is emphasized with A1. The hue is then progressively desaturated from the middle third (A2 with 1 part per 10 parts of orange) at the incisal third (A1 enamel). Therefore, when orange tonality is expressed in the body, it is produced by mixing 1 to 3 parts of orange to 10 parts of dentin.

The enamel distribution (Fig 13–7) should be incorporated in the shade prescription and dictates the amount of reduction of the dentin construction. A

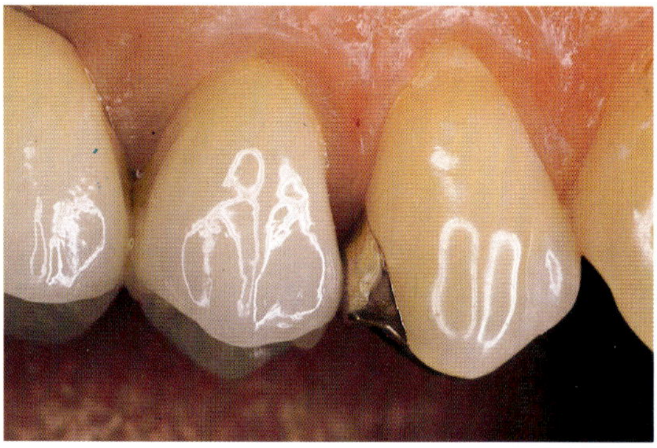

FIG 13–6

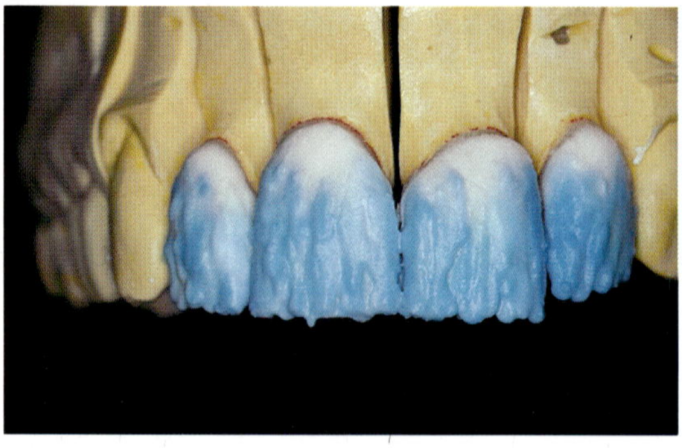

FIG 13–7

progressive fading of the dentin background is more harmonious than abrupt enamel delineation and contrast. Several enamel characteristics are encountered: opalescent enamel is simulated with a mixture of enamel with white and blue and with gray and violet as accessory colors. True opalescent enamel manufactured in some porcelain brands is a true fritted mixture of these ingredients. Semiopaque enamel is a combination of enamel with 10% white and appears to be more dense. It is useful for construction of molars (Figs 13–8 and 13–9). Semitransparent enamel for the incisal edge is an equal mix of enamel with translucent. White opaque enamel spots are only inlaid and combined with up to 70% white.

Variations of enamel translucency induce different patterns of light transmission. Pure enamel can be made to alternate with enamel mixed with 10% white in slightly overlapping narrow vertical bands.

In this maxillary three-unit bridge (Fig 13–10), the longitudinal dentin pro-

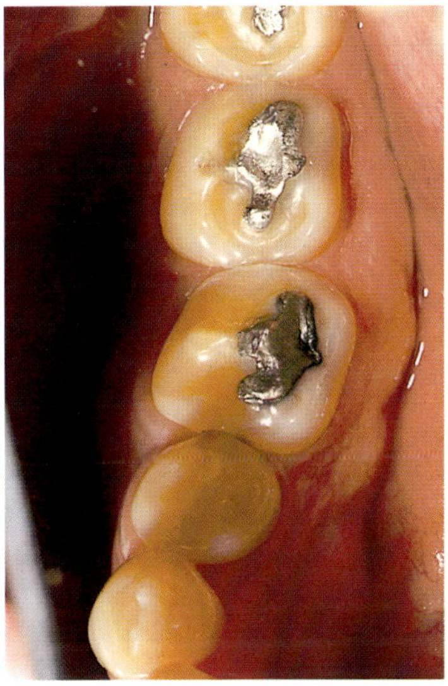

FIG 13–8

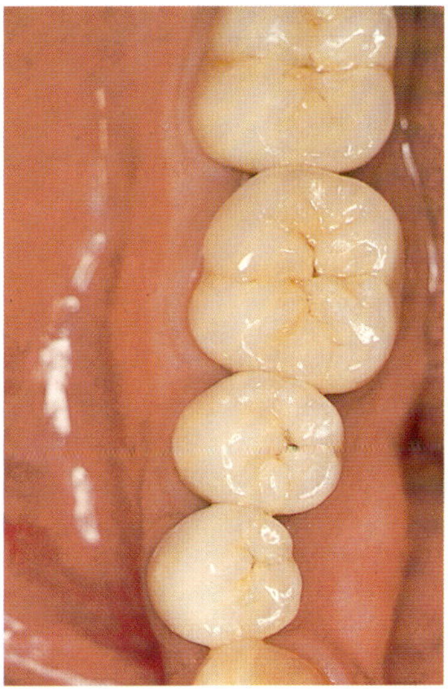

FIG 13–9

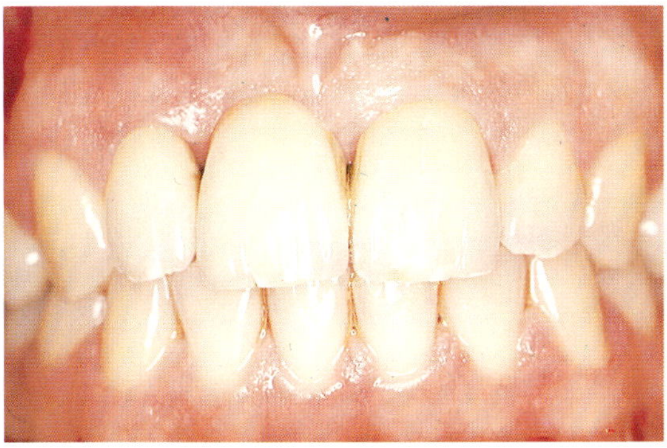

FIG 13–10

gression consists of equal ratios of A1 and A2 in the cervical area, of equal ratios of A2 and A3 with 10% orange in the infrabulge, and A2 in the middle third. The mesiodistal enamel progression over the incisal third consists of several alternations of enamel with 10% white, enamel mixed with translucent, and pure translucent. Scattered opacities in the incisal one third are inlays of pure white and orange with white.

Color variation patterns are also distributed from central incisor to canine. Figure 13–11 shows a preoperative situation resulting from an automobile accident. Figure 13–12 shows the postoperative result: four porcelain jacket crowns

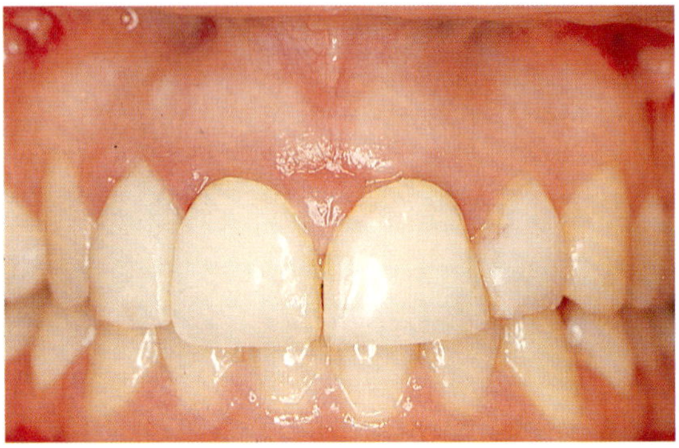

FIG 13–11

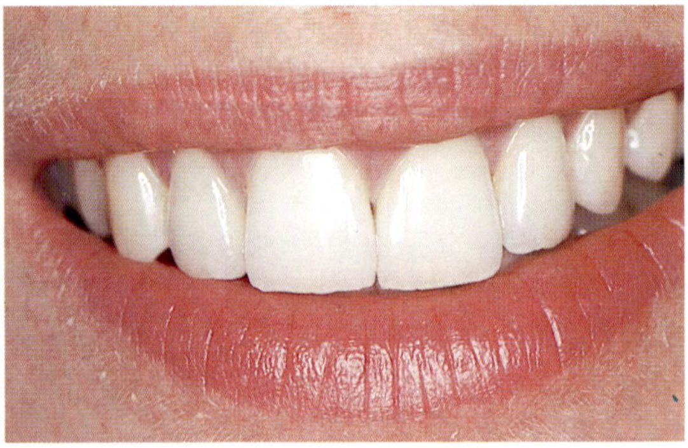

FIG 13–12

constructed for the maxillary incisors. The central incisors are A2, and the lateral incisors are an equal combination of A2 and A3 to achieve a natural progression to the canines, which are A3.

Figure 13–13 illustrates another typical arrangement of four porcelain fused to metal crowns for the maxillary incisors where the central incisors are A2/A3 and the canines are A3/A3.5. The mesial half of the lateral incisors are constructed in A2/A3 and their distal half in A3/A3.5. Slight rotation of the lateral incisors dictates application of opacious dentin[15] in the mesial triangle lingual to the line angles to prevent shadowing in the embrasures. Mechanical polishing of all convexities, after glazing, involves line angles, cervical convexity, and incisal

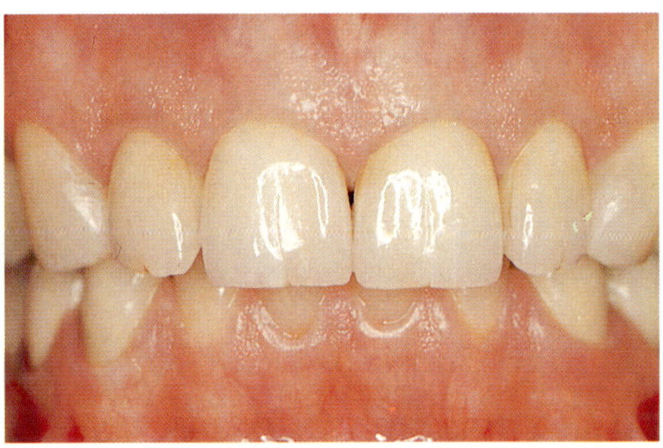

FIG 13–13

edge so that their luster is separately emphasized. Compare the relative dullness of the three-powder constructions with more complex internal effects enhancing depth and vitality and also shifting to an orange tonality. Both restorations in Figures 13–14 to 13–18 incorporate the same minimum amount of surface colorants.

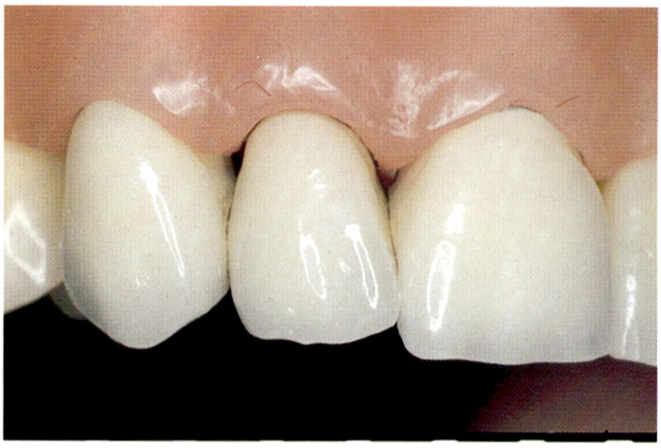

FIG 13–14

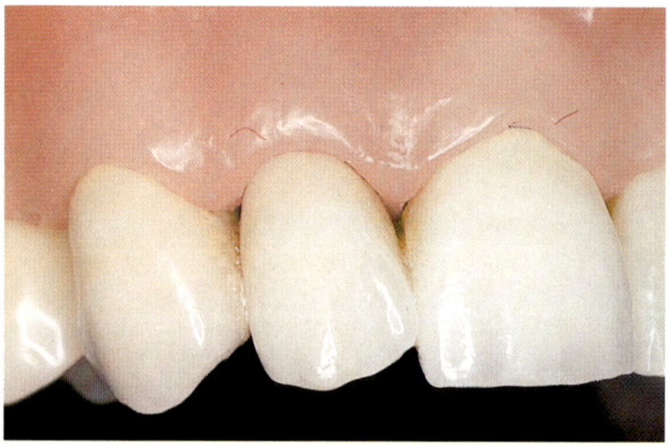

FIG 13–15

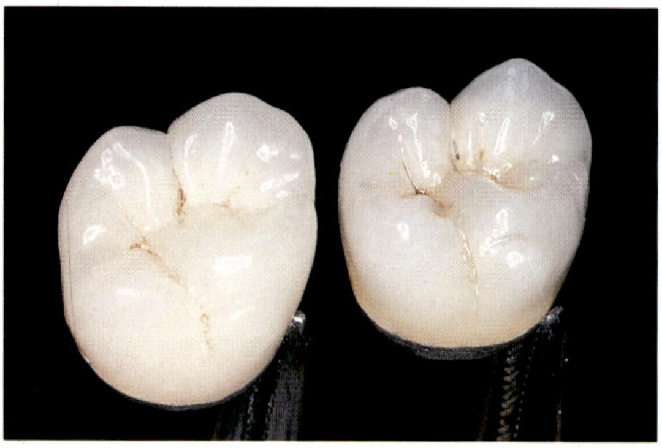

FIG 13–16

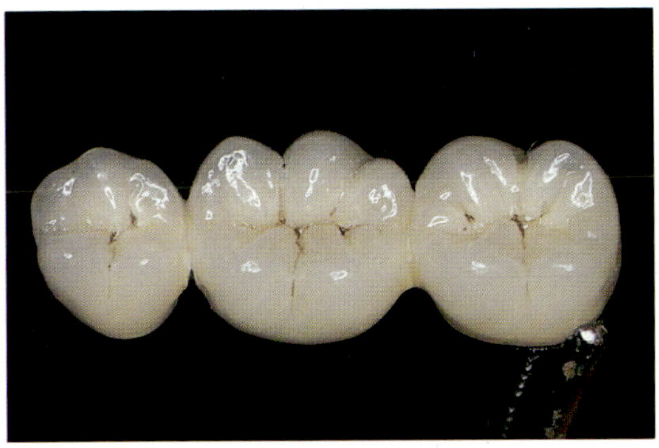

FIG 13–17

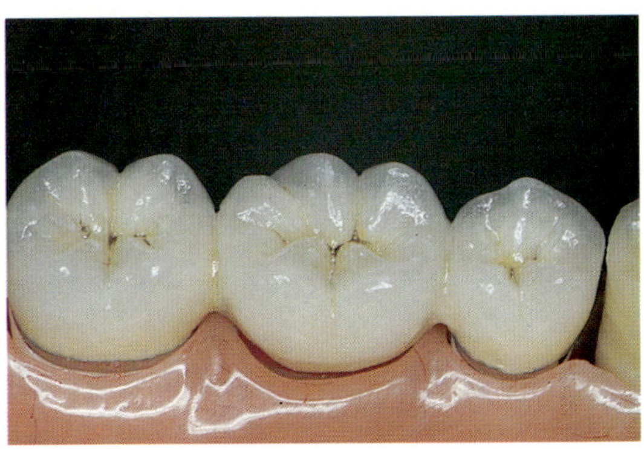

FIG 13–18

SURFACE STAINING

Surface colorants are metal oxides and as such are highly reflective and will decrease translucency when applied over the whole crown surface.[1] They are best utilized sparingly as a finishing touch for slight increase in saturation or densification or for reproducing natural surface characteristics (e.g., tobacco stains, surface decalcifications). They have limited potential to decrease the value of a crown with application of a complementary color to yellow or orange and will often produce, at best, a compromised metameric product. Surface colorants should be used to enhance individuality in the embrasures with dark brown or depth in the occlusal surface. Occlusal staining is a combination involving black in the pits, scattered dark brown over the developmental grooves, and white, especially on the triangular ridge areas bordering the occlusal pit.

This contrasting pattern is effective only on the condition that the accessory grooves be left untouched (Fig 13–19). It is also possible to further emphasize occlusal convexities with diluted white porcelain during enamel construction.

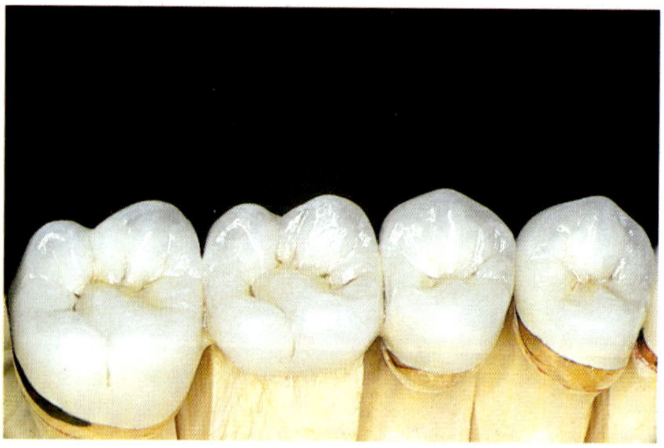

FIG 13–19

REFERENCES

1. McLean JW: *The Science and Art of Dental Ceramics.* Chicago, Quintessence Publishing Co, 1980, vol 2.
2. Yamamoto M: *Metal Ceramics.* Chicago, Quintessence Publishing Co, 1985.
3. Lund TW, Schwabacher WB, Goodkind RJ: Spectrophometric study of the relationship between body porcelain color and applied metallic oxide pigments. *J Prosthet Dent* 1985; 53:790–796.
4. Miller LL, Hemendinger H, in Preston JD, Bergen SF (eds): *Color Science and Dental Art: A Self Teaching Program.* St Louis, CV Mosby Co, 1980.
5. Jorgenson MW, Goodkind RJ: Spectrometric study of five porcelain shades relative to the dimensions of color porcelain thickness and repeated firings. *J Prosthet Dent* 1979; 42:96–105.
6. Preston JD, Bergen SF (eds): *Color Science and Dental Art: A Self Teaching Program.* St Louis, CV Mosby Co, 1980.
7. Clark EB: Tooth color selections. *J Am Dent Assoc* 1933; 20:1065–1073.
8. Hayashi T: *Medical Color Standard: V. Tooth Crown.* Tokyo, Japan Color Institute, 1967.
9. Sproull RC: Color matching in dentistry: II. Practical applications of the organization of color. *J Prosthet Dent* 1973; 29:556–566.
10. Lemire PA, Burk BB: *Color in Dentistry.* Bloomfield, Conn, JM Ney Co, 1975.
11. Geller W: Personal communication, Paris, 1983.
12. Chiche G, Radiguet J, Pinault A, et al: Improved esthetics for the ceramometal crowns. *Int J Periodont Rest Dent* 1986; 1:77–85.
13. Jacobs SH, Goodacre CJ, Moore BK, et al: Effect of porcelain thickness and type of metal ceramic alloy on color. *J Prosthet Dent* 1987; 57:2.
14. Barghi N, Lorenzana RE: Optimum thickness of opaque and body porcelain. *J Prosthet Dent* 1982; 48:429.
15. Geller W: Dark and shadowed zones—an important aspect of the creative shading technique. *Quintessence Dent Technol* 1983; 7:483.

Chapter **14**

Maxillary First Molar: Eight-Powder Construction

When occlusal clearance is minimal and value needs to be lowered significantly, the second opaque layer may be more characterized. Orange opaque modifier applied over the fossa emphasizes depth. Additional contrast is created with violet opaque modifier diluted with white opaque over the cusp elevations. Brown and orange opaque modifiers, respectively, on the proximal and cervical areas increase saturation and depth perspective and generally are the only indicated modifications when occlusal clearance is not critical.

Mix cervical and dentin powders in equal proportions with distilled water, and condense them over the cervical areas so that they are chamfered over the opaque layer. This creates stronger saturation under minimum thickness without surface colorants (Fig 14–1). This effect will be too exaggerated if only pure

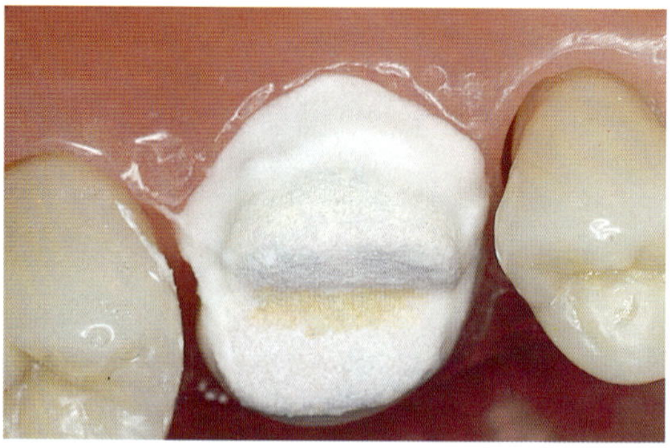

FIG 14–1

cervical porcelain is used. Because calcification increases with age, greater cervical saturation may be necessary. Similarly, cervical intensity is minimal in a young individual. The anatomical contours are built to normal dimensions, into occlusion (see Chapter 5). The cervical convexity is slightly accentuated to compensate for shrinkage. The axial and occlusal reductions follow the sequence described in Chapter 11.

Mix orange powder with distilled water, and paint it over each occlusal pit. Coat the labial developmental groove with an equal mixture of orange and brown porcelains (Fig 14–2).

Mix 12 parts of enamel with 5 parts of blue and 2 parts of white powder in distilled water and proceed to the enamel construction (see Chapter 11) (Fig 14–3).

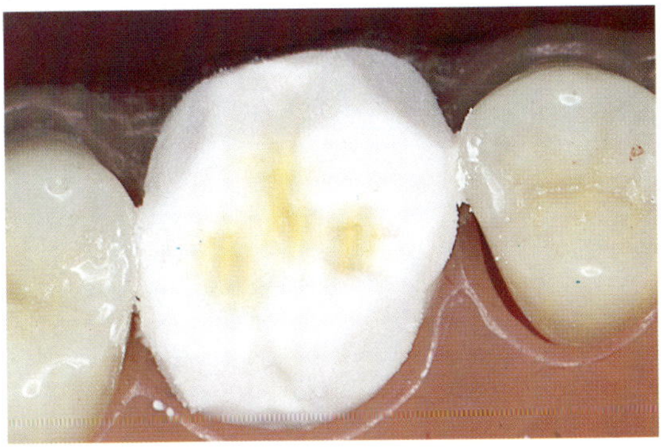

FIG 14–2

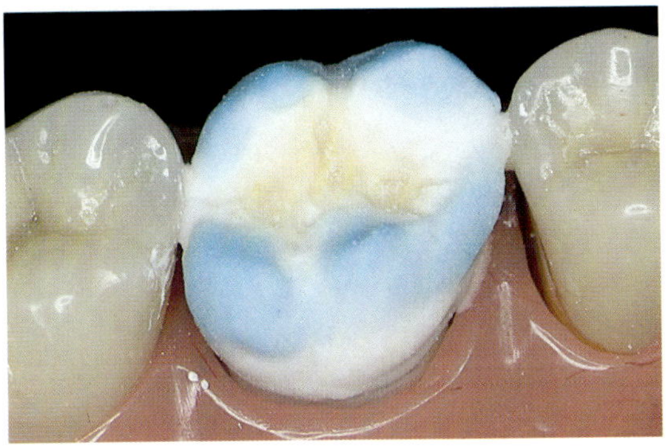

FIG 14–3

Raise the articular pin by 1 mm, and apply the translucent coating (Fig 14–4) in occlusion at the elevated vertical dimension (see Chapter 11).

Mix white powder with distilled water into a very diluted wash, and paint it over the cusp tip and marginal and triangular ridges (green tag in Fig 14–5). This accentuates whitening and elevation perspective.

Enlarge the proximal contacts with enamel covered with translucent porcelain. Apply two separate ultrasonic vibrations of 1 second each, and absorb excess moisture with tissue paper. Deepen the occlusal pits with the point of the grooving blade so that each cusp may shrink separately during firing without tearing the grooves apart.

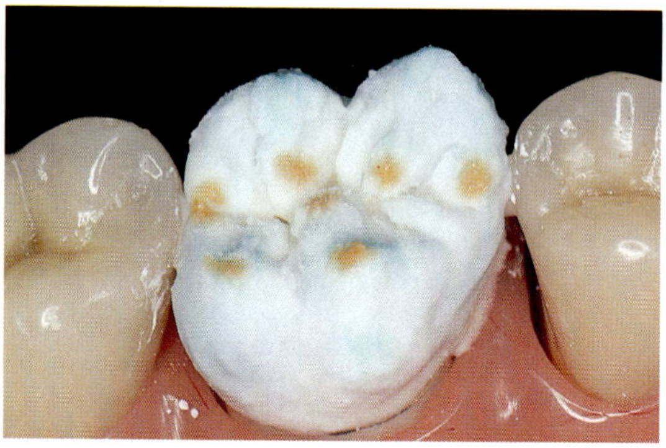

FIG 14–4

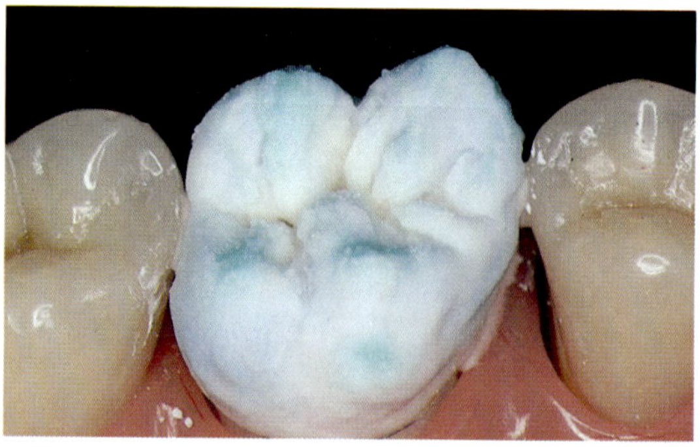

FIG 14–5

After one firing, the lobes and grooves pattern is virtually undisturbed. Color distribution is controlled (Fig 14–6).

Proximal contacts and axial contours are reshaped with tapered diamond burs (Fig 14–7).

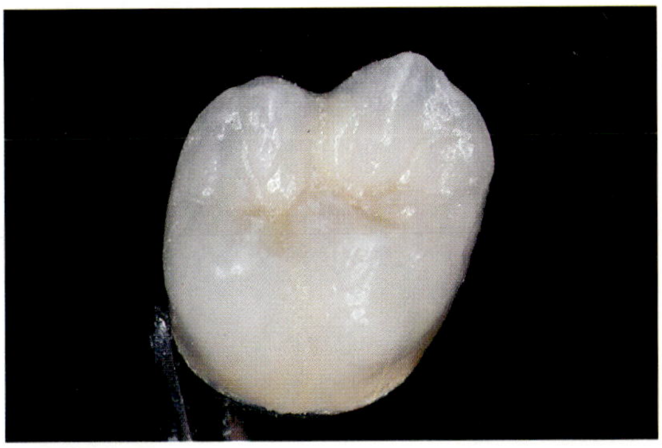

FIG 14–6

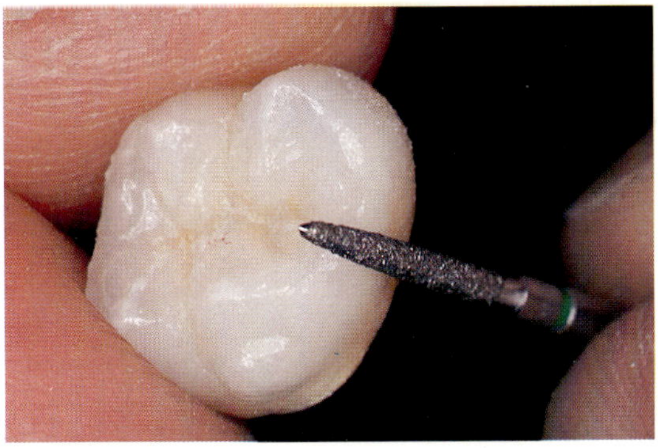

FIG 14–7

Supplemental and developmental grooves are refined with inverted cone and fluted carbide burs (Figs 14–8 and 14–9).

Occlusal interferences are eliminated with a round diamond stone (Fig 14–10). The crown is thoroughly cleaned in ultrasonic solution before surface co-

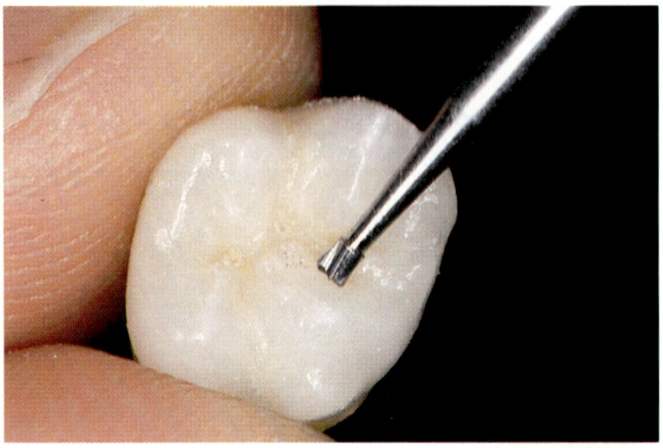

FIG 14–8

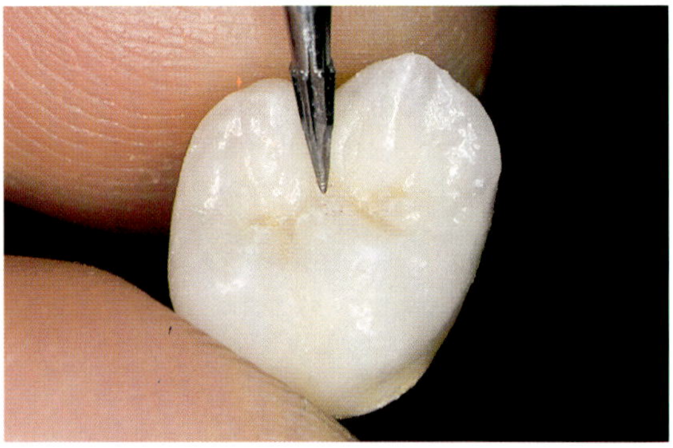

FIG 14–9

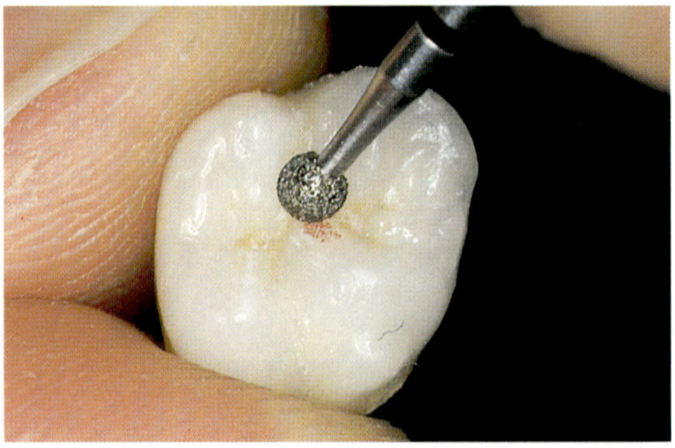

FIG 14–10

lorants are applied; black stain is placed in the occlusal pits, and dark brown stain is scattered along the developmental grooves (Fig 14–11).

Figure 14–12 shows the labial view after glazing; cervical saturation is stronger but remains subtle. Depth illusion is reinforced with contrasting patterns of

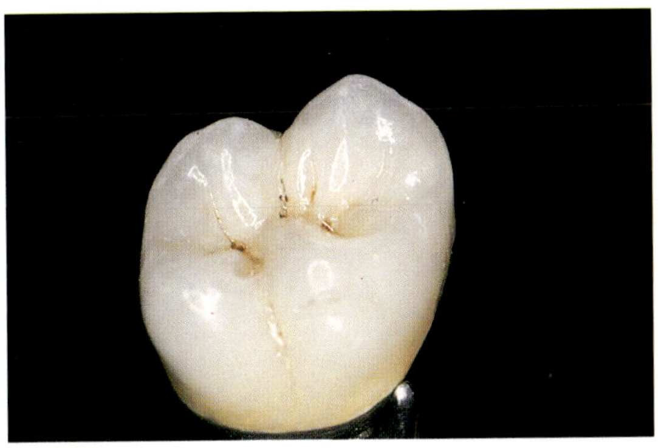

FIG 14–11

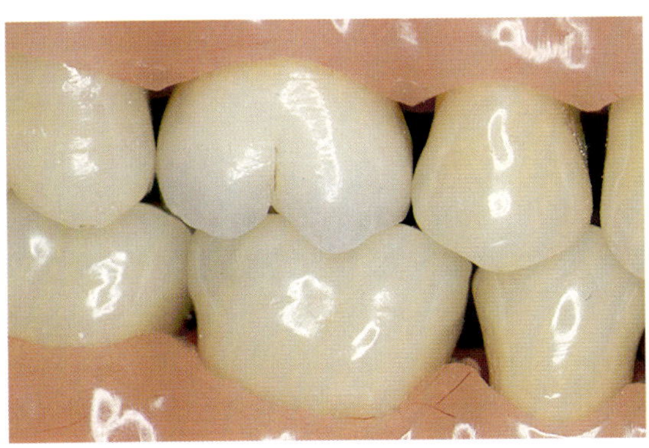

FIG 14–12

internal shade. All depressions are inlaid with orange or brown, and all elevations rely on violet, blue, and white (Fig 14–13). In Figure 14–14, the grooves pattern is under microscopic examination. No tear from cusp shrinkage is detectable.

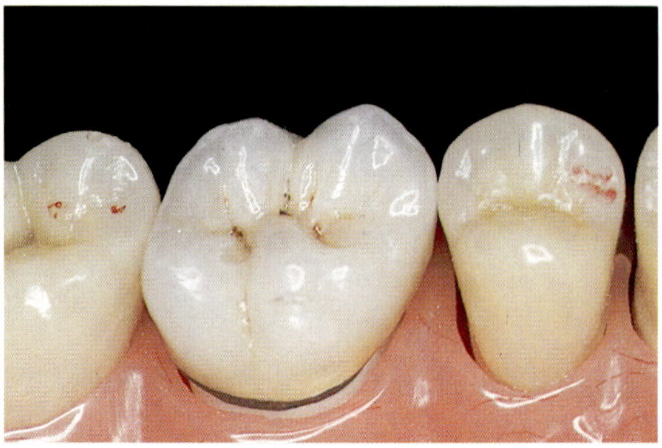

FIG 14–13

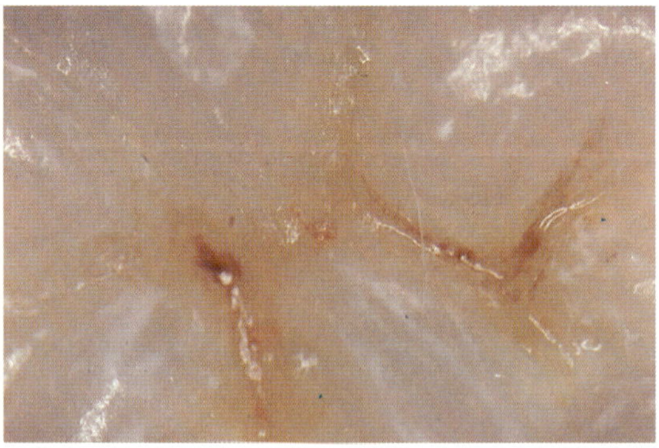

FIG 14–14

Chapter 15

Maxillary Three-Unit Bridge: Ten-Powder Construction

As emphasized before, the precision of the buildup is essential. Do not vibrate during the whole body construction; sharp boundaries must be preserved between each layer. Opaque characterization may be useful when value needs to be decreased or when the space allocated for porcelain is minimal. Cervical saturation and embrasure depth are emphasized with orange and brown and orange opaque modifiers, respectively. Violet opaque modifier over the incisal third portions serves to lower value and also mimic opalescence. This area is critical in terms of potential for show-through of opaque (Fig 15–1).

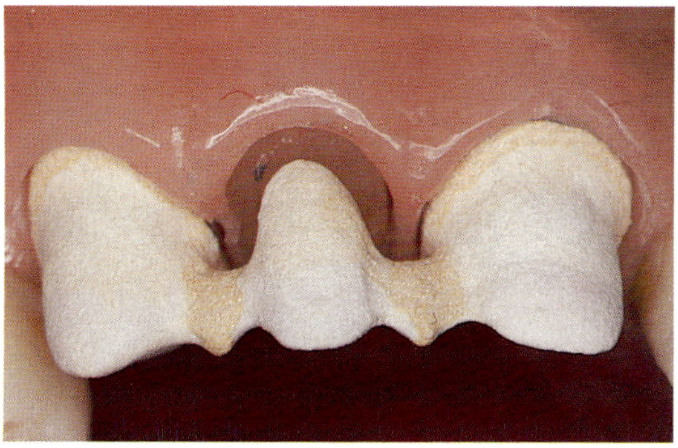

FIG 15–1

After the opaques are fired, a very thin coating of opacious dentin is layered over the whole framework (Fig 15–2). It should be slightly thicker cervically and extend incisally 1 mm beyond the opaque level for subtle enamel progression. Opacious dentin is a very efficient transitional background since a minimum section is sufficient to neutralize opaque reflectivity and still allow for adequate dentin thickness for shade reproduction. It also prevents shadowing and graying at the interproximal embrasures.

Mix two parts of orange powder with eight parts of dentin in distilled water, and condense them in the cervical region (Fig 15–3). The shade prescription often dictates an orange cervical hue. This is the most obvious area in which to express redness in the tooth.

A natural color progression must be created from the central incisor to the canine. For example, when the central incisor is an equal mix of A2 and A3 shades and the canine is A3.5, the lateral incisor shade should be A3.

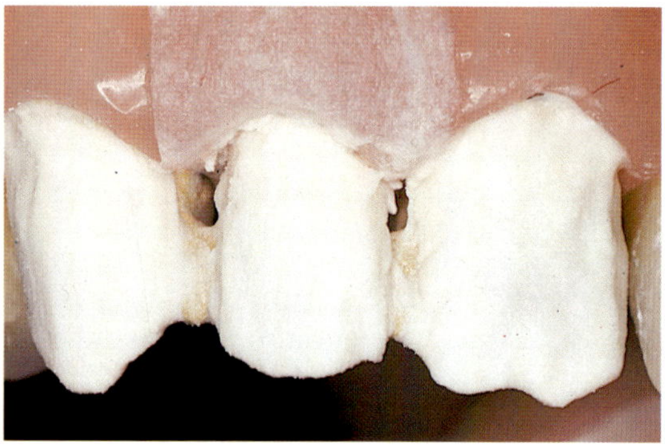

FIG 15–2

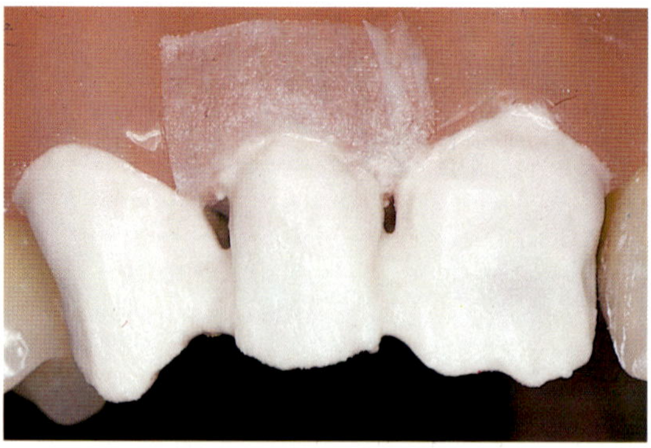

FIG 15–3

Another typical arrangement from A2 on the central incisor to A3.5 on the canine is to construct the mesial half of the lateral incisor with A2 and its distal half with A3.5. These patterns, which are indicated to prevent uniformity from one unit to the other, are produced in the dentin buildup only (see Chapter 6). All anatomical contours are built to normal dimensions (Fig 15–4). Extend the incisal edges by 1 mm, and slightly accentuate the line angles and the cervical convexities to compensate for shrinkage. Reduce the incisal third of the central incisor, the labial two thirds of the lateral incisor, and the labial half of the canine. Coat the embrasures and the lingual concavities with orange porcelain. Further prepare the central incisor for incisal mamelons and the lateral incisor for a wavy incisal effect (Fig 15–5). The lingual reductions are also performed at this stage (see Chapter 11).

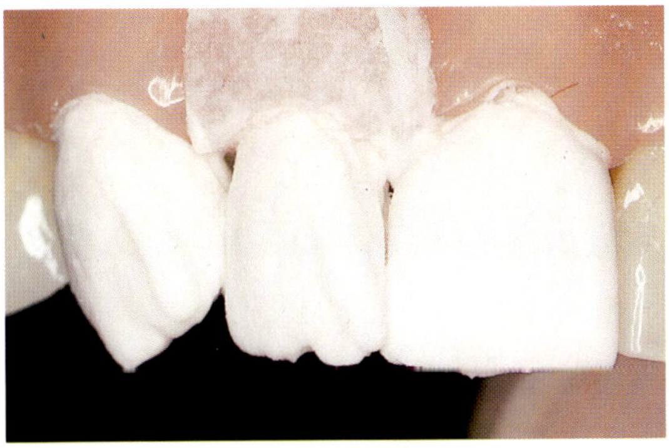

FIG 15–4

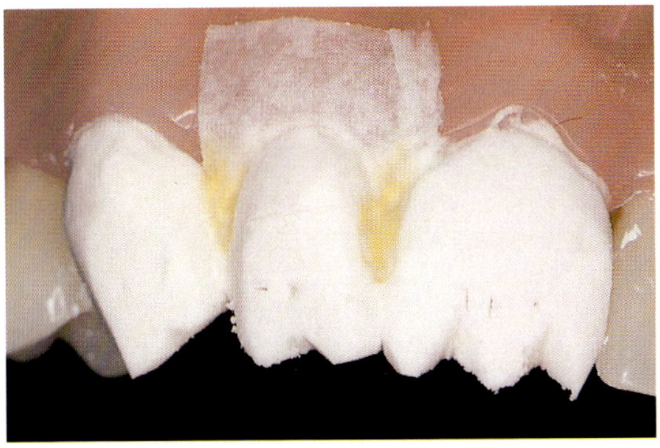

FIG 15–5

Emphasize the dentin enamel contrast by creating a concavity in each fingered extension and in the lateral incisal groove, and apply a combination of one part of yellow opaque modifier with three parts of light brown dentin (Fig 15–6). Soften these characterizations with a dentin overlay. All internal effects must remain subtle (Fig 15–7).

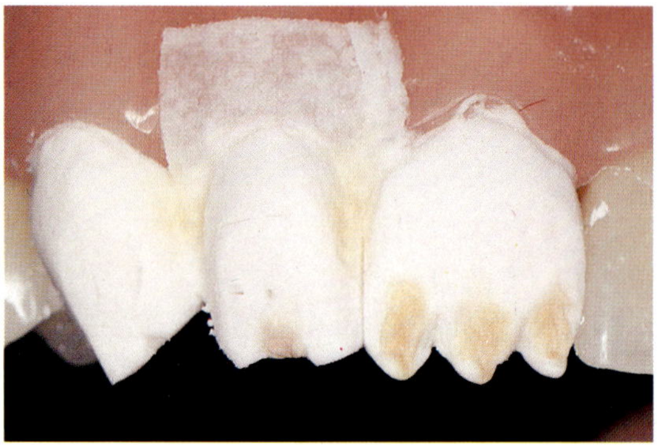

FIG 15–6

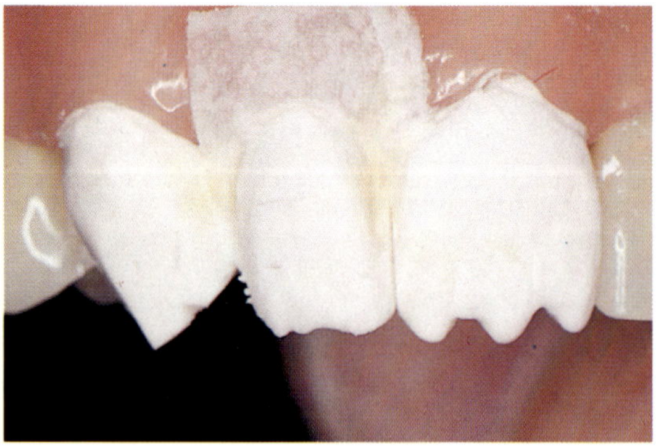

FIG 15–7

Carve two horizontal grooves in each labial surface. Restore them with a mixture of the lightest dentin of the A range (A1) with 10% white (green tag). These bands emphasize convexity and produce interspersed opacity (Fig. 15–8).

The enamel construction also contributes in breaking uniformity in translucency by promoting subtle color variations and additional refraction. Start covering the mesial line angle of the central incisor with a 1–mm wide longitudinal strip of enamel (blue tag). Then alternate overlapping strips of enamel mixed with 10% white (violet tag) with pure enamel strips (Fig 15–9). Progress in a

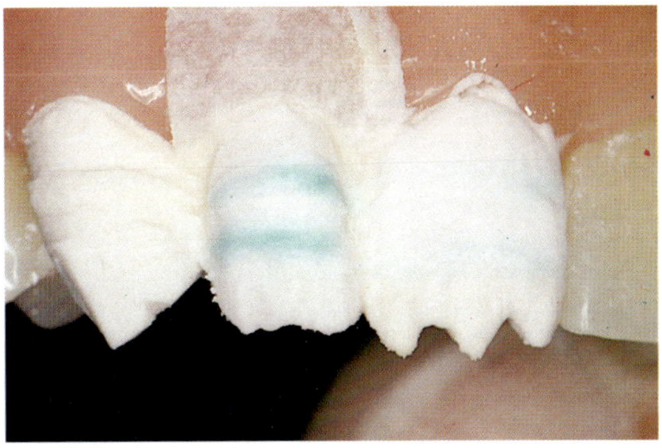

FIG 15–8

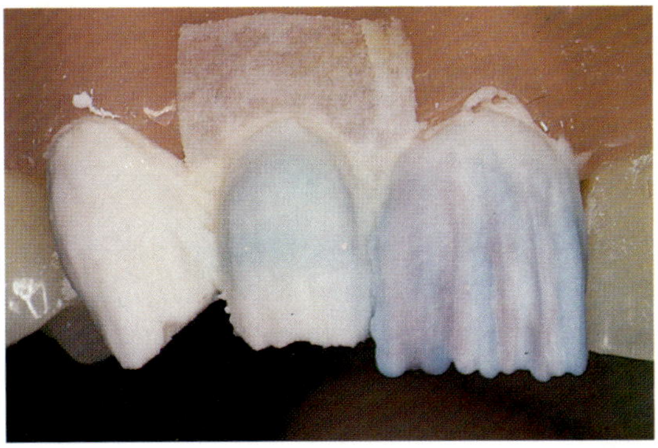

FIG 15–9

mesiodistal direction to the canine (Fig 15–10). The incisal edges remain 1 mm longer than normal (see Chapter 11). The lingual ridges are restored with enamel but are still kept out of occlusion when possible.

Raise the incisal pin by 1 mm. Apply the translucent overlay (see Chapter 11). Emphasize lobes and line angles to compensate for shrinkage. This coating is no thicker than 0.2 to 0.3 mm; otherwise the value will be lowered more than necessary (Fig 15–11). Restore the lingual contours into occlusion with translucent procelain (Fig 15–12). Apply two separate ultrasonic vibrations of 1 second

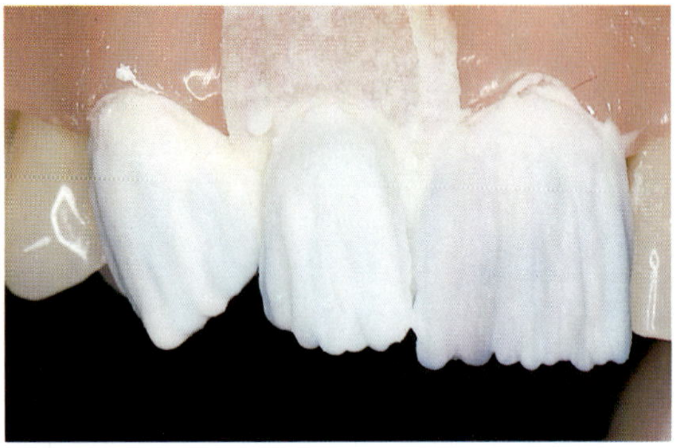

FIG 15–10

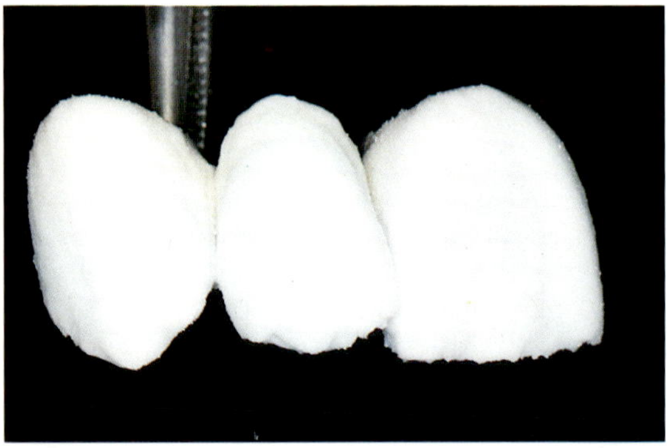

FIG 15–11

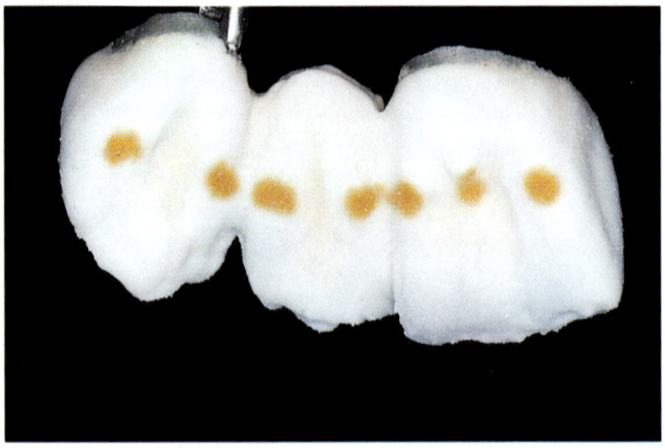

FIG 15–12

each, and absorb excess water with tissue paper.

Predrying time is 9 minutes.

After first firing, color distribution and outlines are controlled. Shrinkage is significant (Fig 15–13).

After reshaping, restore the cervical contours with an equal mix of dentin and translucent, the line angles and marginal ridges with an equal mix of enamel and translucent, and the most superficial areas with translucent (Fig 15–14).

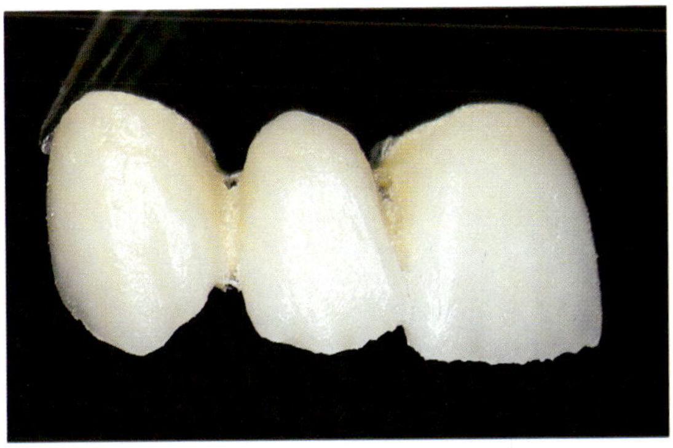

FIG 15–13

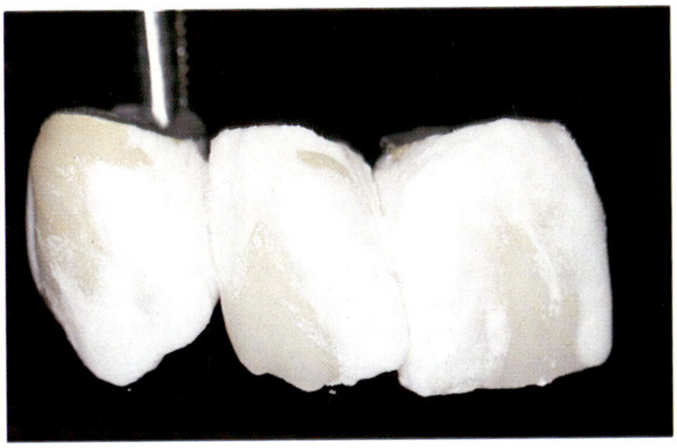

FIG 15–14

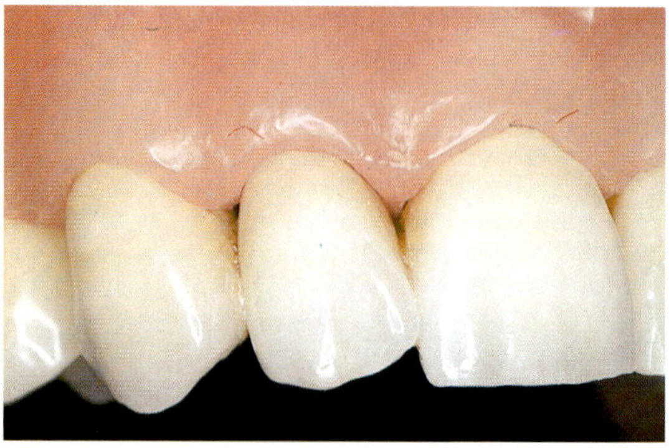

FIG 15–15

The second firing temperature and rate are reduced by 15°C and 10°C, respectively. After firing, refine the contours (see Chapter 9), and thoroughly clean the bridge in ultrasonic solution. Apply light brown surface colorant in the embrasures to accentuate illusion of depth and individuality. Do not use any other surface colorants.

Figure 15–15 shows the completed bridge after glazing. The cervical value is controlled by the modified opaque, the opacious dentin, and the orange saturation. Internal effects remain barely discernible.

Chapter 16

Mandibular Three-Unit Bridge: Ten-Powder Construction

Opaque characterization may be useful when value needs to be decreased, especially for a posterior bridge when the allocated space for porcelain is minimal.

Violet opaque modifier diluted with white modifier is applied over the occlusal and the cusp elevations. Besides reducing value, this reinforces the opalescence of the enamel.

Brown opaque modifier in the embrasures and the buccal developmental grooves serves to emphasize depth. Orange modifier creates saturation and depth at the margins (Fig 16–1).

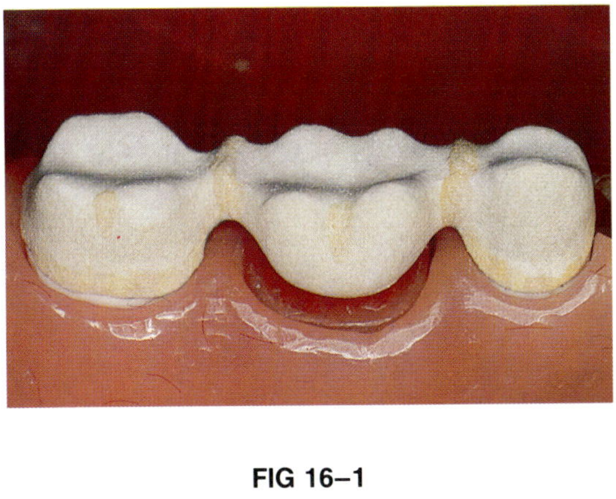

FIG 16–1

After the opaques are fired, a very thin coat of opacious dentin (Fig 16–2) is layered over the whole framework except for the deepest aspect of the embrasures and the center of the connections. It should be slightly thicker cervically and extend above each cusp and over their labial aspect (Fig 16–3). If the opacious dentin does not match the prescribed shade, it is selected as close to it as possible and mixed in equal proportions with dentin before application.

Mix 2 parts of orange powder with 8 parts of dentin, and condense them over the cervical region (Fig 16–4). The shade prescription often dictates a strong cervical hue. This is the most obvious area from which redness is expressed. Cervical powder mixed with dentin may also be indicated as another alternative as prescribed clinically.

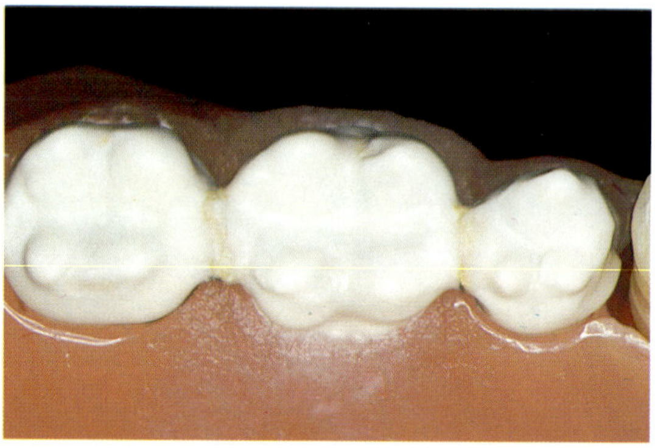

FIG 16–2

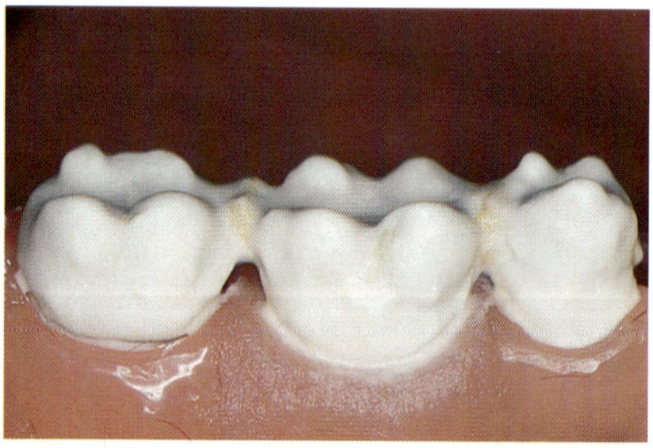

FIG 16–3

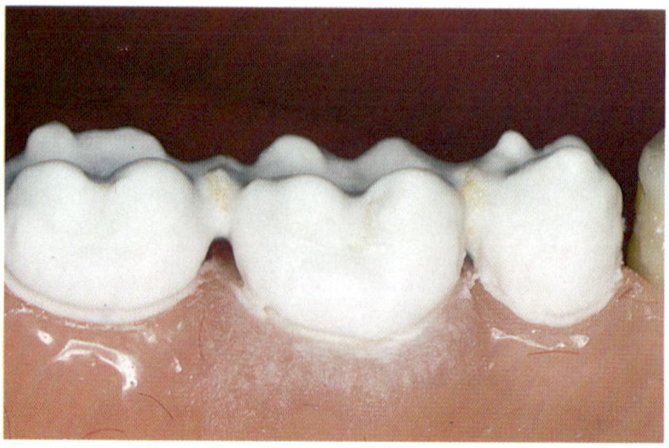

FIG 16–4

Coat the embrasures with orange porcelain for depth (Fig 16–5), and build anatomical contours in dentin (Fig 16–6) to normal dimensions (see Chapter 6). The cervical regions are slightly oversized to compensate for shrinkage.

The axial and occlusal reductions follow the sequence described in Chapter 11. Mix orange powder with distilled water, and paint it over the occlusal developmental grooves. Coat the labial and lingual developmental grooves with an equal combination of orange with brown (Fig 16–7).

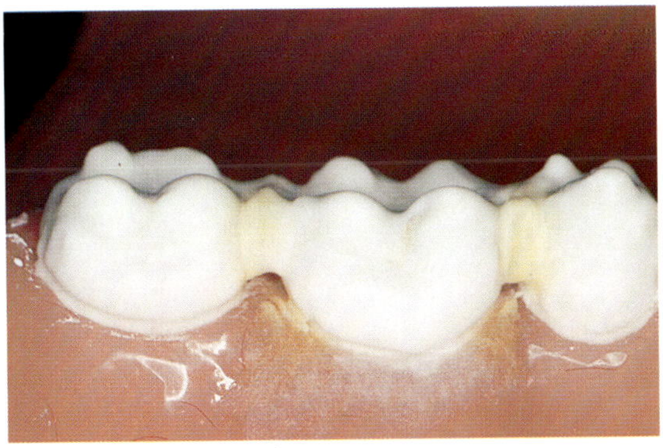

FIG 16–5

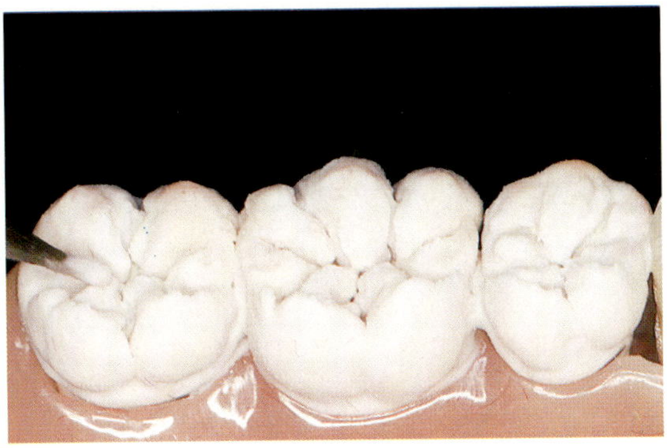

FIG 16–6

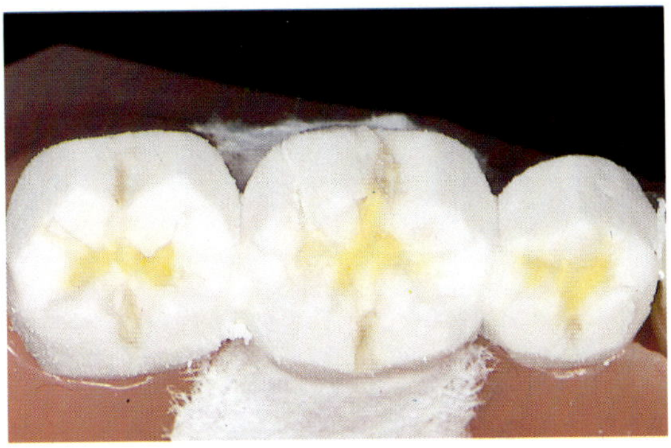

FIG 16–7

Reduce the cervical suprabulges (Fig 16–8), and restore them with the lightest dentin shade of the selected range (A1 in this instance). This enhances the illusion of convexity in this area (Fig 16–9).

Mix 12 parts of enamel with 5 parts of blue and 2 parts of white powder, and proceed to the enamel construction (see Chapter 12). Only the centric cusps should be in occlusion at this stage (Fig 16–10). Elevate the articulator pin by 1

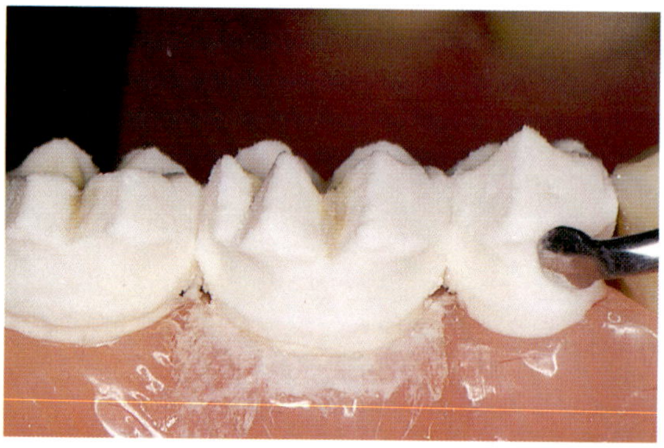

FIG 16–8

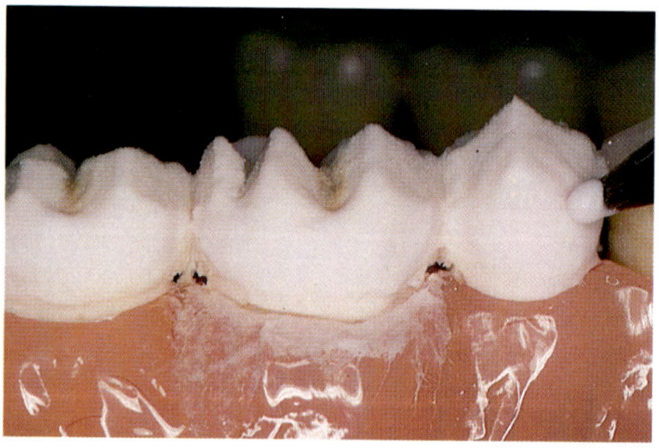

FIG 16–9

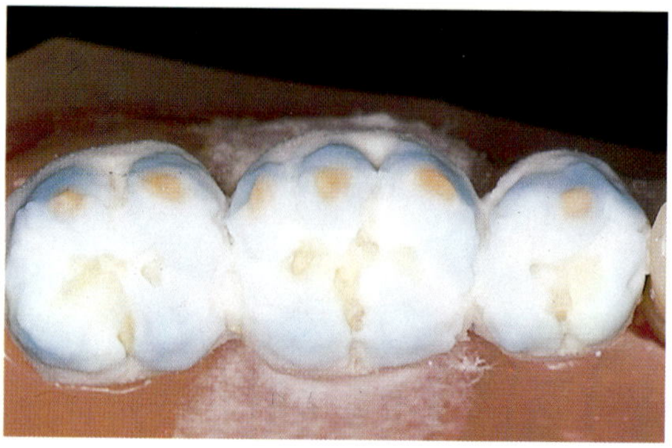

FIG 16–10

mm. Apply the translucent overlay (Fig 16–11) (see Chapter 12). Check the occlusion for major interferences (Fig 16–12). Be careful not to detach or break the buildup from its base.

Finish and polish the axial contours with the large soft-hair brush. Refine the developmental and supplemental grooves with the tip of the fine sable-hair brush. Lightly polish the occlusal surfaces with the large soft-hair brush. Apply two separate ultrasonic vibrations of 1 second each, and absorb the excess moisture with tissue paper. Deepen the occlusal pits with the point of the grooving blade so that each cusp shrinks separately during firing without tearing the grooves apart. Enlarge the proximal contacts with enamel covered with translucent porcelain. Refine the underside of the pontic into a modified ridge lap design.

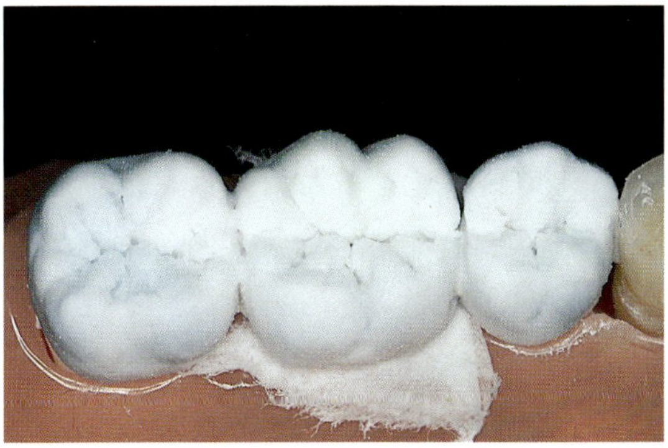

FIG 16–11

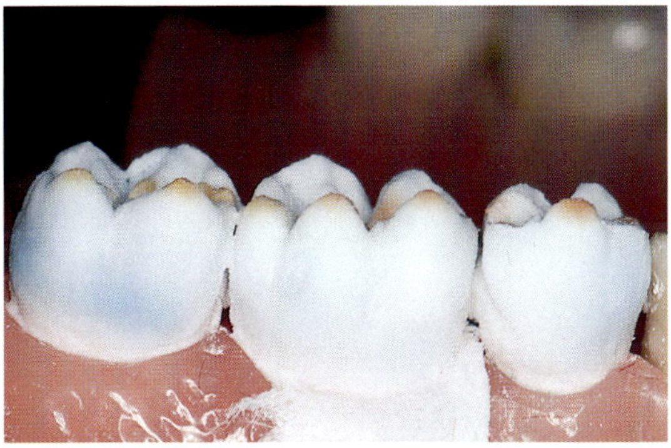

FIG 16–12

Predry the bridge over the firing tray for 9 minutes (Fig 16–13). After first firing, shrinkage is significant, but outlines and color distribution are preserved (Fig 16–14).

Additions are made with dentin and translucent mixed in equal parts over the cervical third, enamel and translucent mixed in equal parts over the middle third, and translucent over the incisal third and the occlusal surface. Any missing occlusal contact is restored in this phase.

The second firing is performed at a reduced temperature (−15°C) and increased firing rate (10°C).

After firing, the anatomy needs to be refined but not recreated. Finishing is accomplished with diamond stones and carbide burs (see Chapter 14). The ridge and groove pattern needs only minimum alterations. Occlusal prematurities are adjusted until harmonious occlusion is achieved (Fig 16–15). Clean the bridge thoroughly in ultrasonic solution. Figure 16–16 shows the completed bridge after glazing. An equal mix of black and brown surface colorants was applied in the occlusal pits and dark brown scattered along the developmental grooves and the embrasures. Cervical saturation is stronger but subtle and imparts a redder tone to the construction. Translucency is not compromised with surface colorants (Fig 16–17).

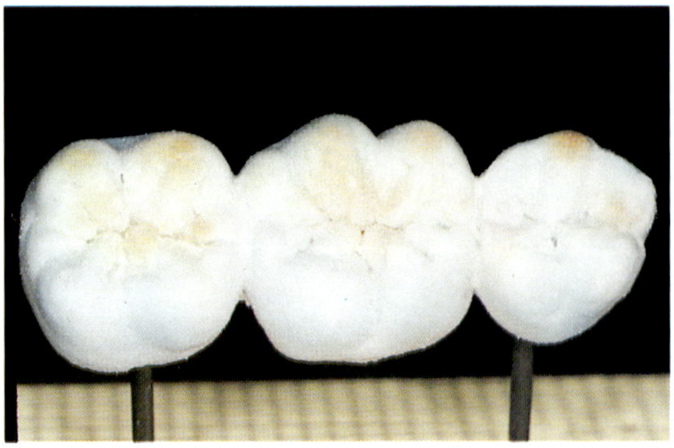

FIG 16–13

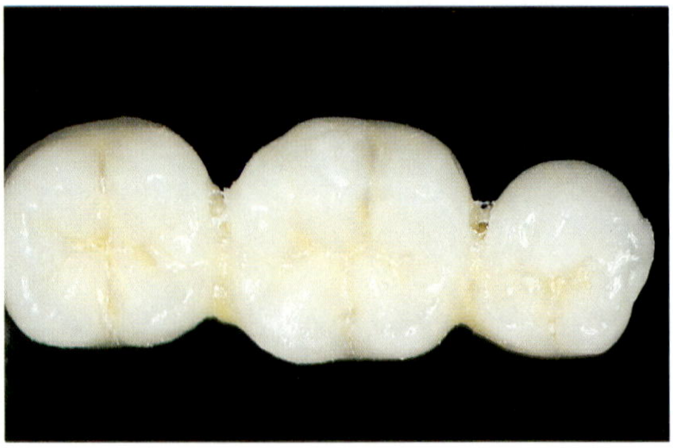

FIG 16–14

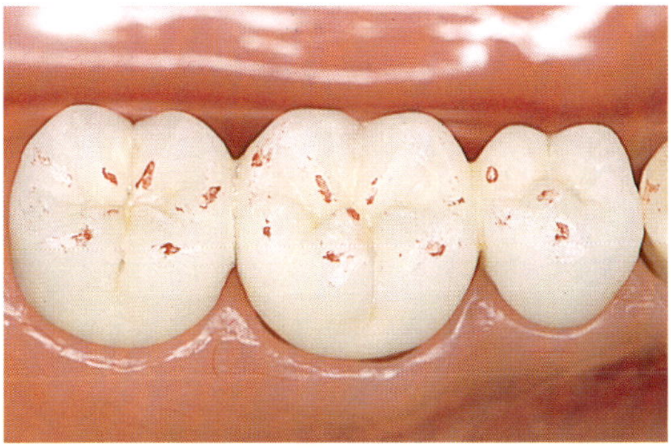

FIG 16–15

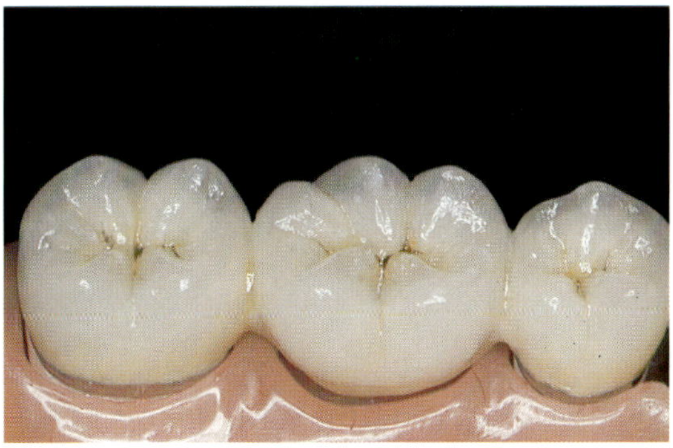

FIG 16–16

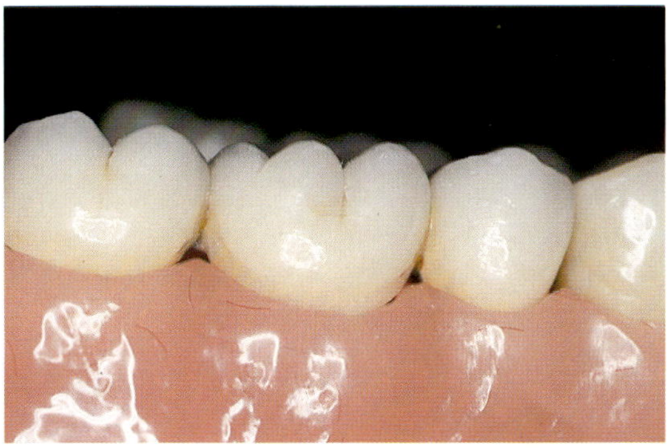

FIG 16–17

Chapter 17

Esthetic Margin Techniques

PORCELAIN MARGINS

Porcelain margins provide the most esthetic design; they eliminate the liability of metal margins but are also weaker because they are unsupported. A 1.2– to 1.5–mm wide shoulder preparation with internally rounded angle at 90 to 100 degrees to the root surface is recommended. It creates maximum bulk of porcelain at its edge and is most resistant to tensile stresses. Smoothness is essential; a corrugated finish line results in porcelain irregularities that are more prone to fracture, especially at clinical try-in.[1] The tissue protecting end (TPE) diamond bur (Fig 17–1) produces a very smooth surface without damage to the marginal periodontium or any undercuts in the axial wall of the preparation because of its smooth beveled side.[2]

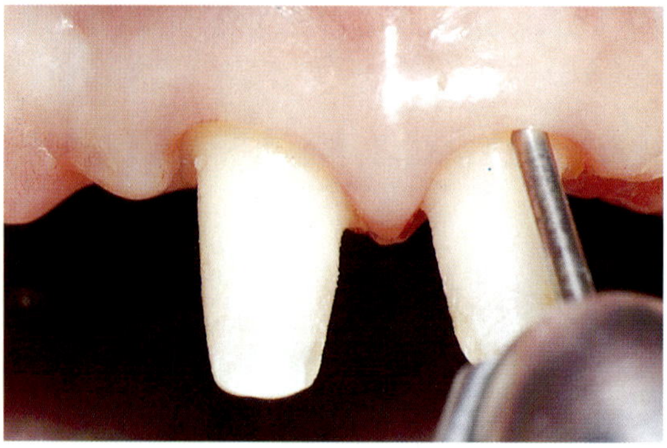

FIG 17–1

Numerous techniques of porcelain margin construction using platinum matrix, refractory dies, or separating varnish have been advocated.[3–8] Their respective performances vary with operator skill and are dissimilar in terms of marginal adaptation and reproduction, resistance to pyroplastic flow, and surface quality.[9, 10] Translucency may also be compromised since the body porcelain is subjected to additional firings to secure marginal adaptation. The edge of this porcelain margin is slightly rounded, and a large porosity is detectable (Fig 17–2).

In our experience, the shoulder porcelain method yields the best results. It does not require advanced skills, is easy to master, and is easy to integrate within any laboratory protocol. Marginal adaptation with adequate cervical hue can be routinely achieved in two firings. All porcelain margin techniques require additional firings, the exception here being that the body porcelain is constructed only after marginal adaptation is finalized, and it will be subjected only to its regular firing cycle and will preserve its translucency. Good marginal fit is still maintained[11] after glazing, and surface texture is homogeneous under light microscopic examination (Fig 17–3). When the shoulder angle exceeds 100 degrees,

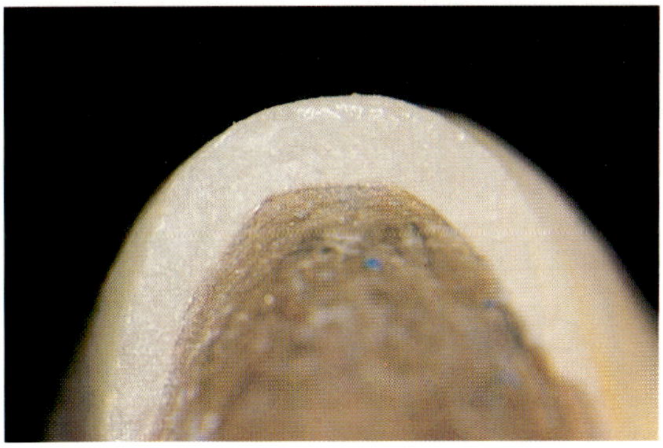

FIG 17–2

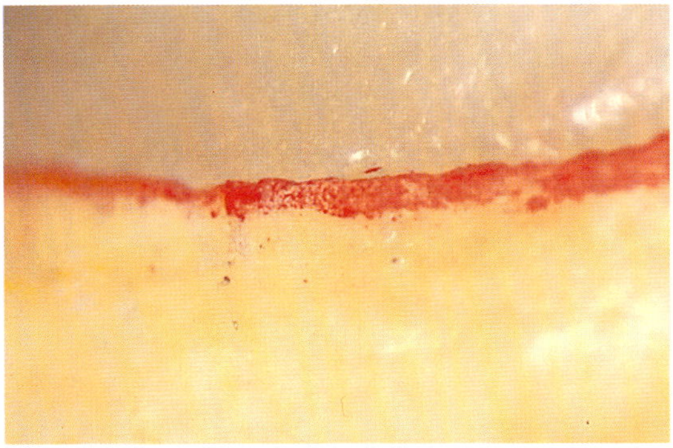

FIG 17–3

the porcelain becomes thinner at the labial edge unless it is overcontoured and is more vulnerable to chipping (Fig 17–4). The steeper the shoulder angle, the more shrinkage at the margin and lack of adaptation. In periodontal situations where the shoulder angle and thickness are unfavorable, a hairline metal collar is a preferred alternative when the finish lines extend well into the cement area (Fig 17–5).

A clinical retrospective study by the authors conducted with J. Radiguet, D.D.S., and P. Genini, C.D.T., involving 191 units identically constructed with shoulder porcelain margins demonstrates the reliability of this technique when precautions are observed (Table 17–1).

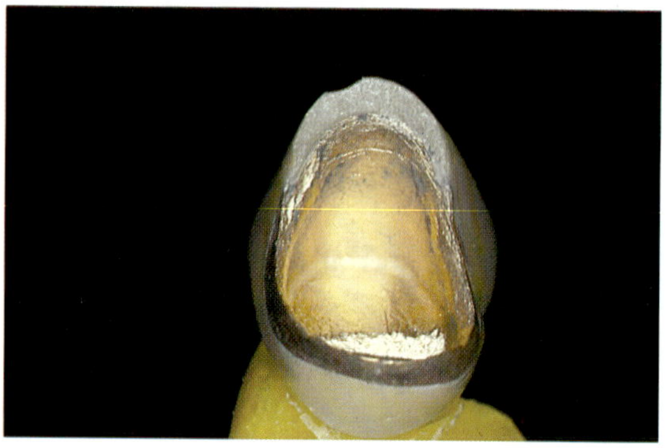

FIG 17–4

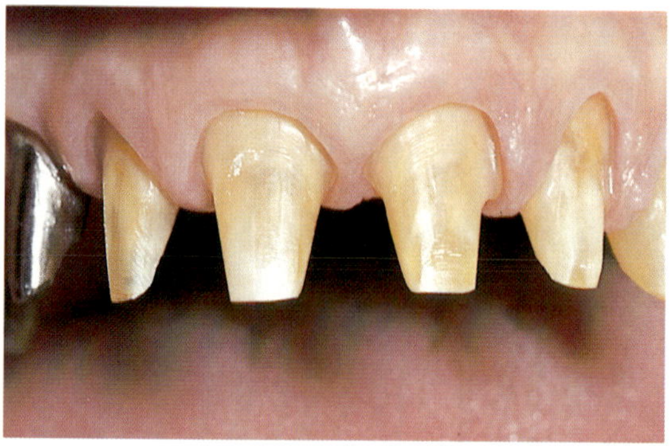

FIG 17–5

TABLE 17–1.
Results of Clinical Testing of Shoulder Porcelains

Yr	Total no. of Crowns	Single Units	Bridge Abutments	No. of Fractures	Anterior Location	Posterior Location
1983	5	5			4	1
1984	45	40	5	1*	25	20
1985	69	51	18	2*	28	41
1986	72	51	21	1†	39	33
Total	191	147‡	44§	4	96	95

*Bridge abutment.
†Single unit.
‡66 anterior and 81 posterior locations.
§30 anterior and 14 posterior locations.

Single Units.—The labial metal collar is eliminated from the shoulder and is horizontally beveled along the proximal aspects to provide for a progressive overlap of porcelain on metal (Fig 17–6). For optimum cervical depth of translucency, the opaque layer is kept along the axial walls and does not extend onto the shoulder. Lubricate the die with a porcelain-release agent (Fig 17–7). Apply

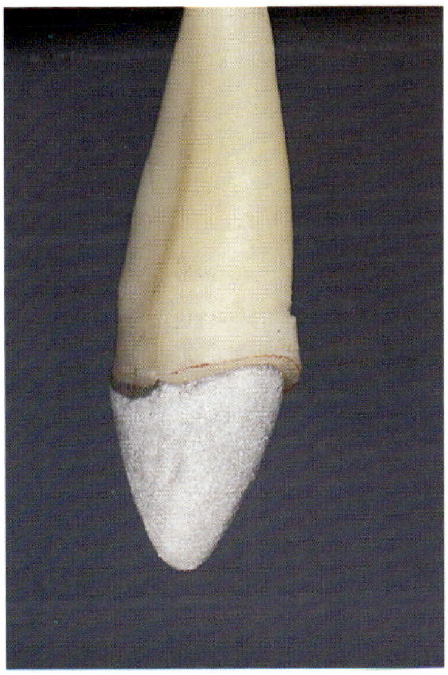

FIG 17–6

FIG 17–7

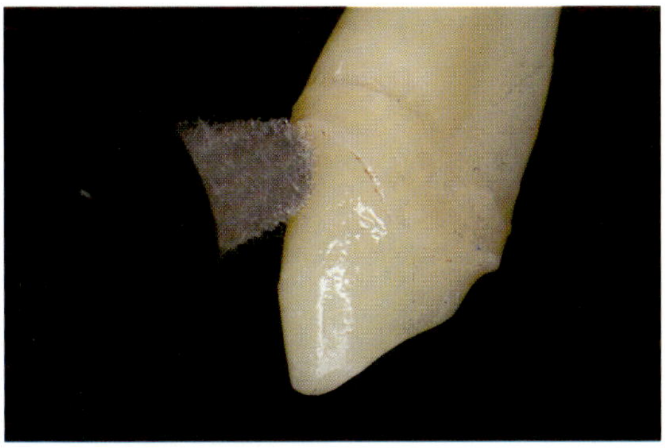

a small bead of shoulder porcelain of the selected shade at the mesiolabial line angle (Fig 17–8), and spread it along the margin using light pressure on the brush. Its teardrop configuration is chamfered over the opaque (Fig 17–9). Apply three separate ultrasonic vibrations of 1 second each. These bring the shoulder porcelain into closer adaptation to the margin (Fig 17–10). Absorb the excess

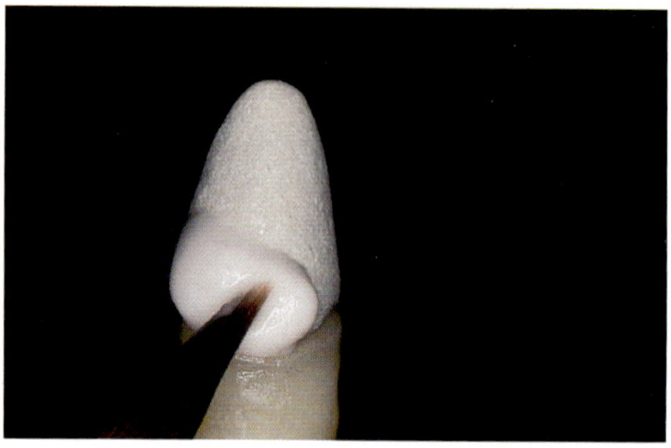

FIG 17–8

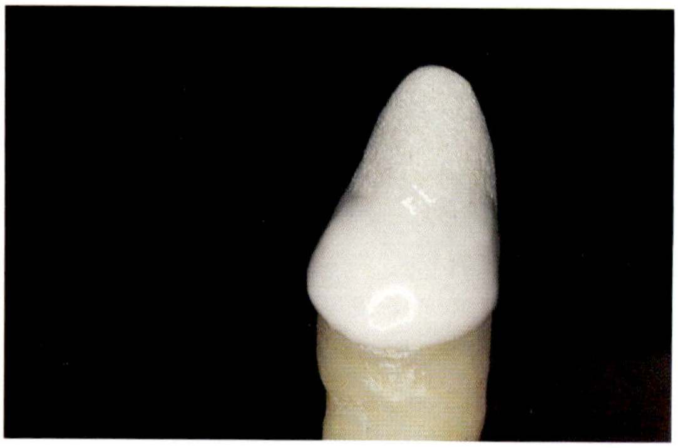

FIG 17–9

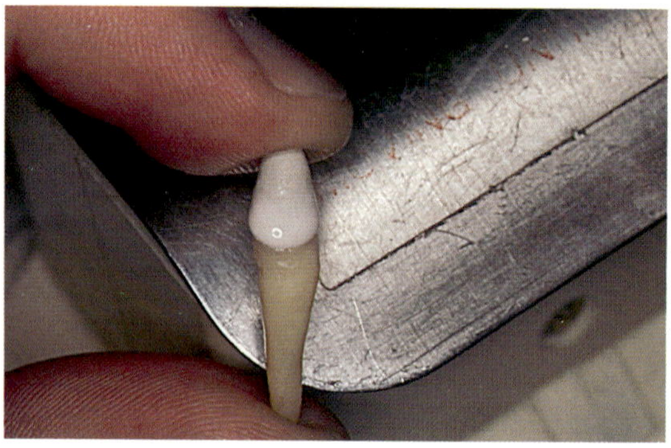

FIG 17–10

water with tissue paper. Maintain the crown firmly in position with finger pressure, and burnish the condensed mix. Flush with the edge of the margin with the large soft-hair brush in vertical downward strokes only (Fig 17–11). Dust off any excess with lateral sweeps. Carefully lift the crown from the die with a steady controlled pressure of the fingertips pushing against one another (Fig 17–12). Do not attempt to seat the crown back before firing.

The firing temperature of shoulder porcelains is typically 20°C to 30°C higher than the regular body. For this reason they do not undergo significant distortion during body firing and glazing as long as they are shaped to be covered with a thin layer of porcelain during body construction. If the shoulder porcelain was undercontoured at this stage, it could be lifted during firing of a thicker body layer and would not fuse to it as easily. A typical cervical gap results from

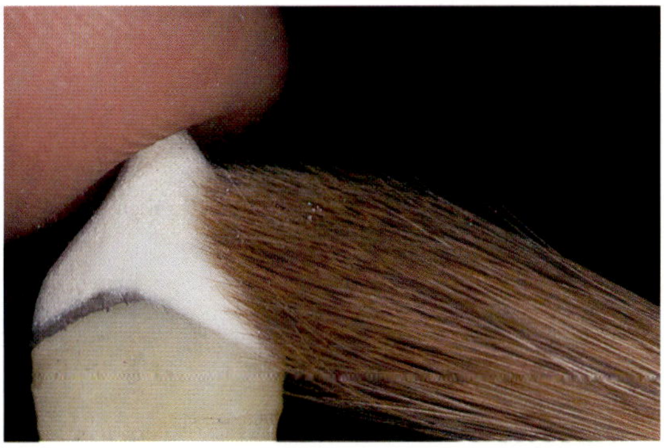

FIG 17–11

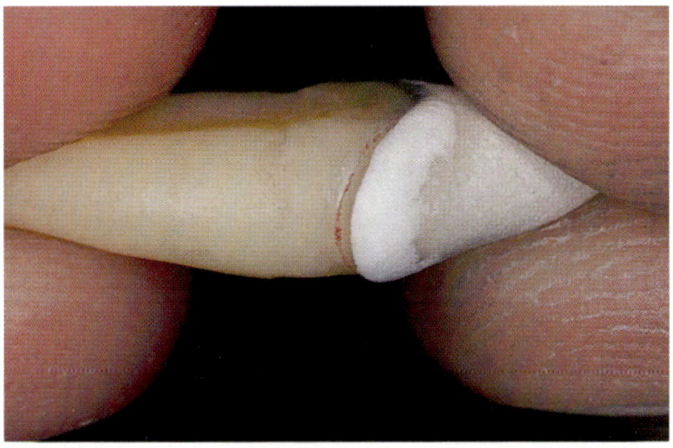

FIG 17–12

shrinkage after the first firing (Fig 17–13). A wash of shoulder porcelain is crushed with a pestle to refine and improve its flow (Fig 17–14). It is flowed into the gap with the crown firmly held into position. Since it is very diluted, water can seep readily to the internal line angle, and when a more saturated increment is applied, it is drawn by capillary action through the whole cervical gap (Fig 17–15). Complete the adaptation with ultrasonic vibrations and polish-

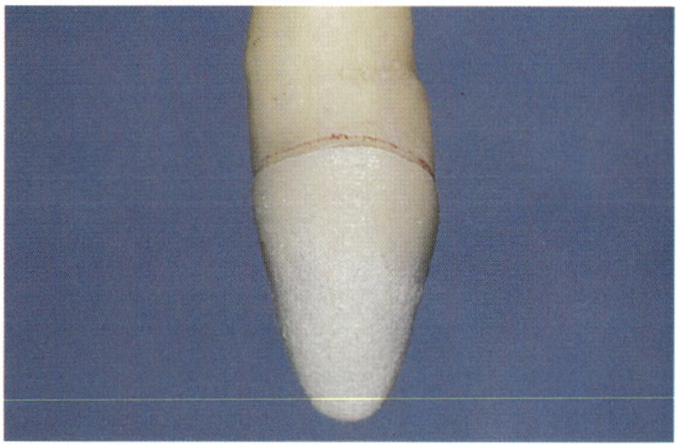

FIG 17–13

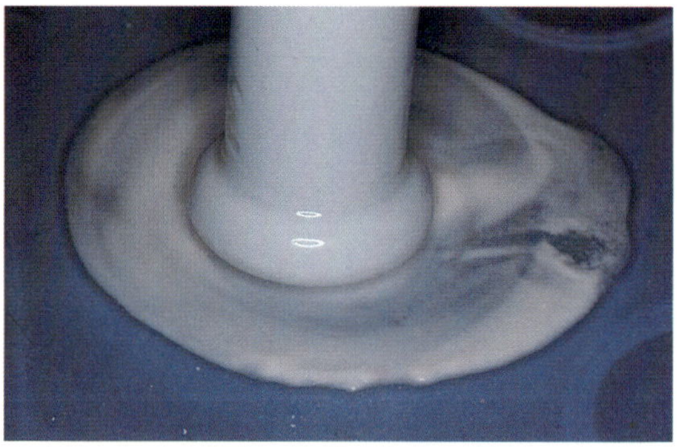

FIG 17–14

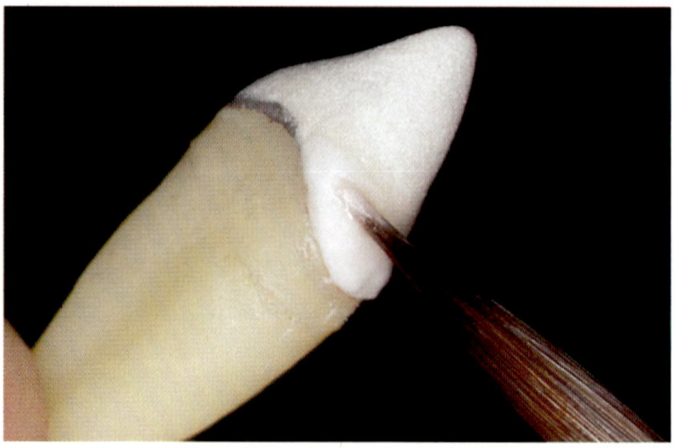

FIG 17–15

ing with the large soft-hair brush, as described earlier (Fig 17–16). The packing density at this step allows for a direct lift-off without deformation, even though metal support is absent, and for negligible shrinkage on firing (Fig 17–17). Complete elimination of shrinkage is theoretically impossible; however, a carefully controlled procedure yields clinically acceptable results. Second firing temperature is reduced by 10°C to 15°C.

The body porcelain is completed and fired. Progress from medium to fine high-speed diamonds when recontouring and finishing the cervical area. The finished crown in Figure 17–18 has acceptable marginal adaptation and translucency.

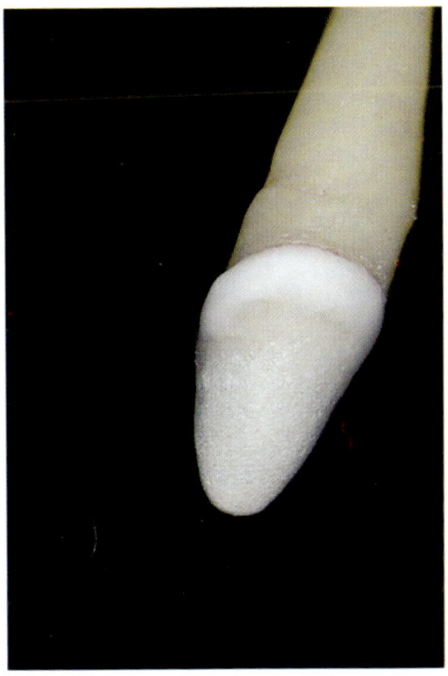

FIG 17–16

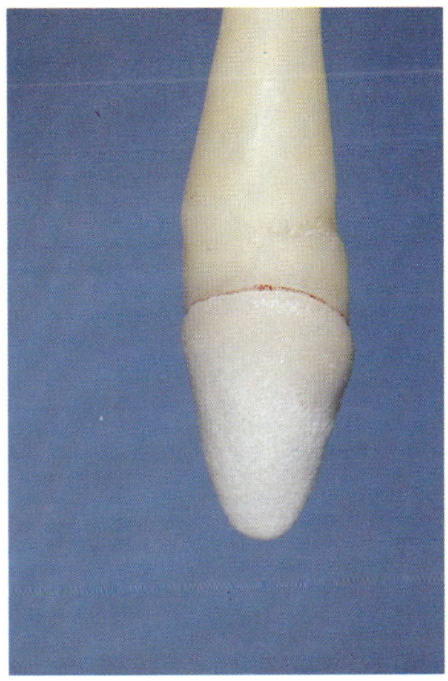

FIG 17–17

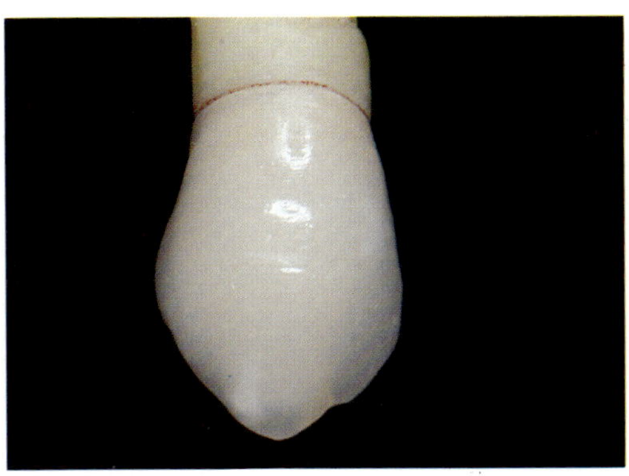

FIG 17–18

Bridge Abutments.—Framework distortion during firing of a well-fitting three-unit bridge may become significant when internal stresses accumulated during grinding and finishing the casting are released. As long as the framework is waxed to its final configuration so that metal preparation is kept to the strictest minimum, distortion of a three-unit bridge remains negligible when casting stresses are eliminated with a preliminary heat treatment. This treatment is performed for 1 hour at a temperature of 100°C below the solidus-liquidus point of the metal, with the casting sprue still connected to the bridge. When porcelain margins are prescribed for both abutments, they must be constructed and vibrated simultaneously (Fig 17–19). The bridge is very precisely separated from the model along its path of draw (Fig 17–20). Cervical corrections after the first

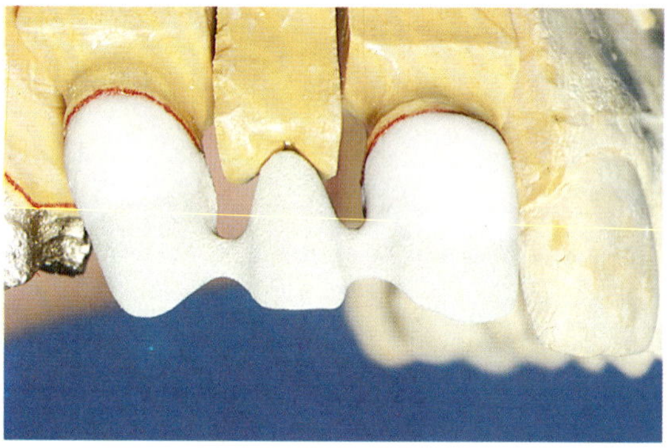

FIG 17–19

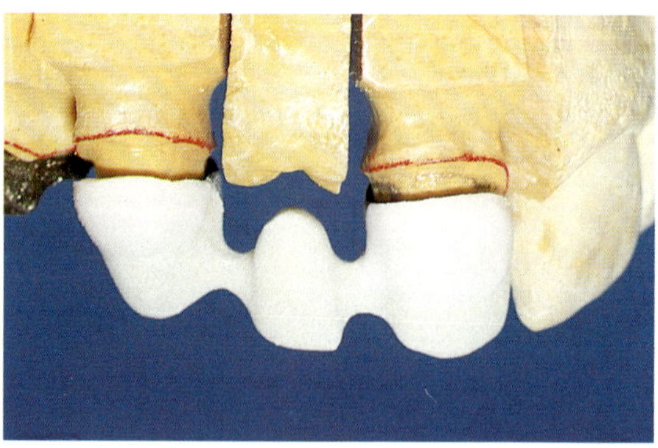

FIG 17–20

firing are performed simultaneously. Final margins are completed in two firings (Fig 17–21). The clinical result: two three-unit bridges restoring the maxillary quadrant. Porcelain margins have been constructed on all four abutments (Fig 17–22). For bridges of greater magnitude, especially a typical maxillary six-unit anterior bridge, framework distortion during firing becomes significant[12] and is difficult to control because of porcelain shrinkage and metal stress release. This is further aggravated by the incorporation of porcelain margins that require two additional firings. It is recommended as a general rule to construct (Fig 17–23)

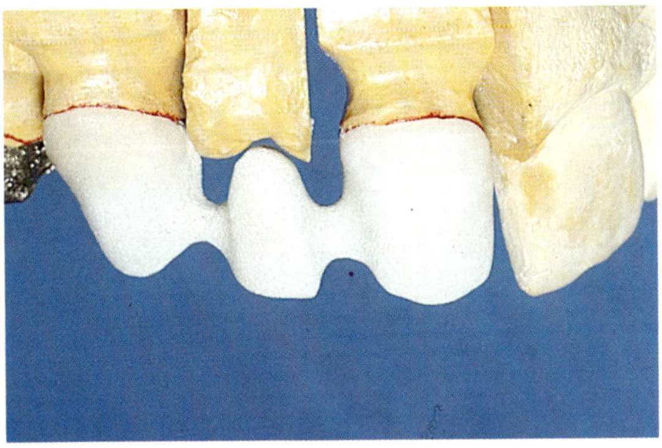

FIG 17–21

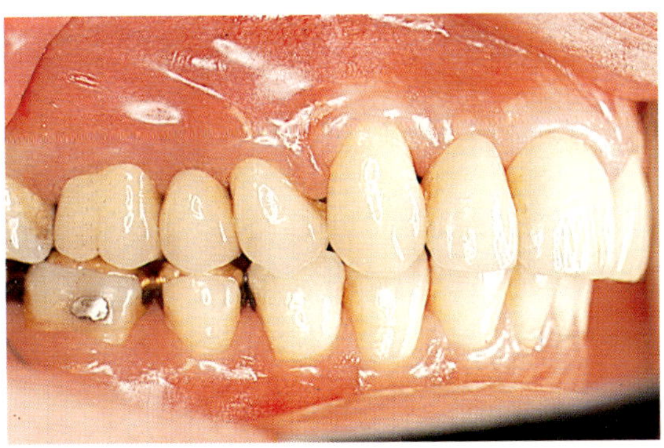

FIG 17–22

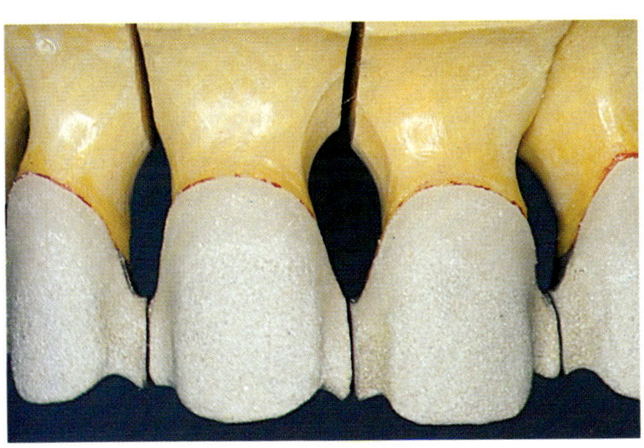

FIG 17–23

and glaze separately, as a single unit first, any porcelain margin retainer and to reunite the fragmented restoration with postceramic soldering (Fig 17–24). Another similar situation is depicted in Figures 17–25 and 17–26.

Porcelain margins may be indicated for any single unit or bridge abutment in the esthetic zone to maximize cervical depth of translucency and esthetics, especially wherever thin marginal gingival tissues may be prone to recession.

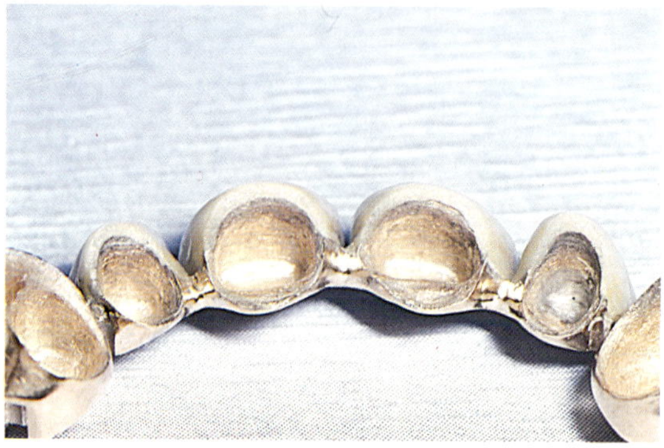

FIG 17–24

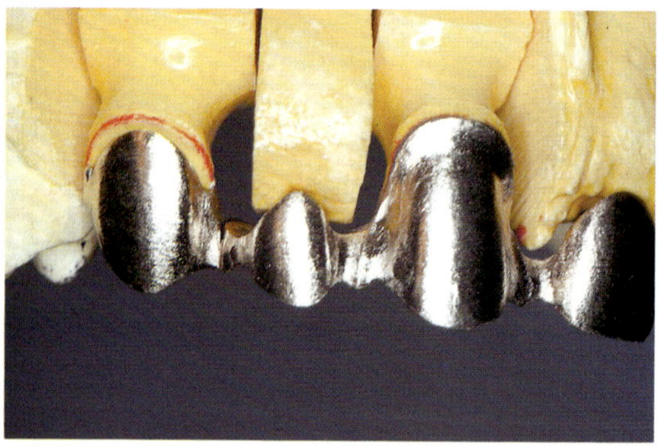

FIG 17–25

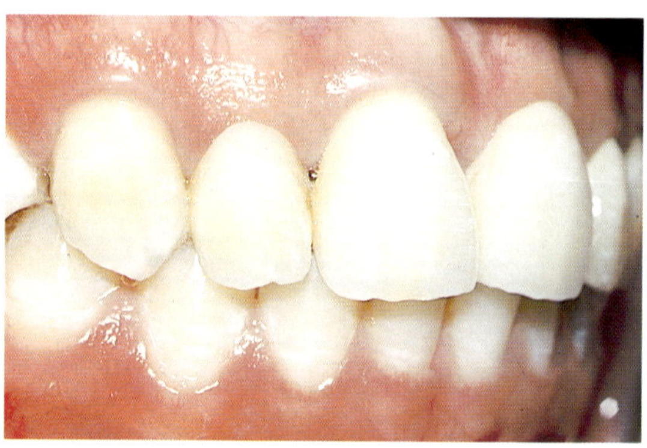

FIG 17–26

However, to prevent any breakage or chipping, they should be strictly limited to situations where all three criteria of shoulder angulation, thickness, and smoothness are met to create an adequate butt joint of porcelain (Fig 17–27). Practically, the esthetic zone involves up to the second premolars (Fig 17–28).

The ideal indication of a porcelain margin bridge is the replacement of the

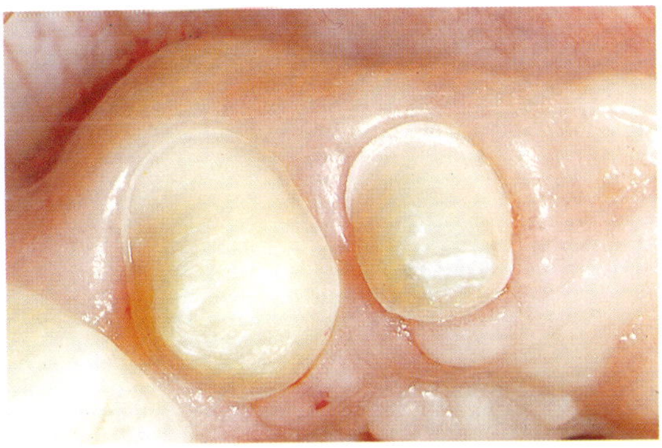

FIG 17–27

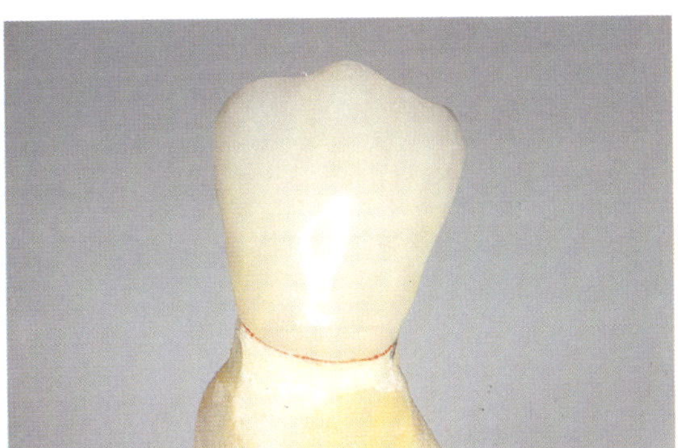

FIG 17–28

maxillary central or lateral incisor or both (Figs 17–29 to 17–31). This is the most esthetic and durable option available when acid-etched bonded retainers are contraindicated.

Porcelain margins may typically chip during clinical try-in if they are subjected to any concentrated wedging, fulcruming, or tensile stress. These are created when a bridge is slightly unstable over the preparations (due to faulty impression, imprecise indexing, or poor temporization), excessive friction is generated (due to insufficient internal relief on the die), or a porcelain margin bridge is cemented temporarily and loosens prematurely or has to be removed with excessive force.[1]

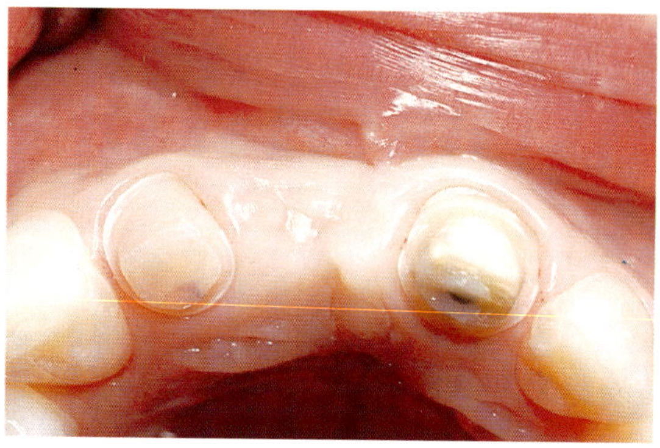

FIG 17–29

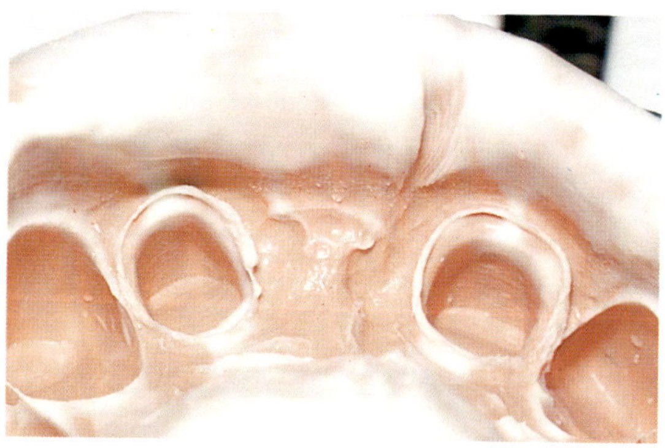

FIG 17–30

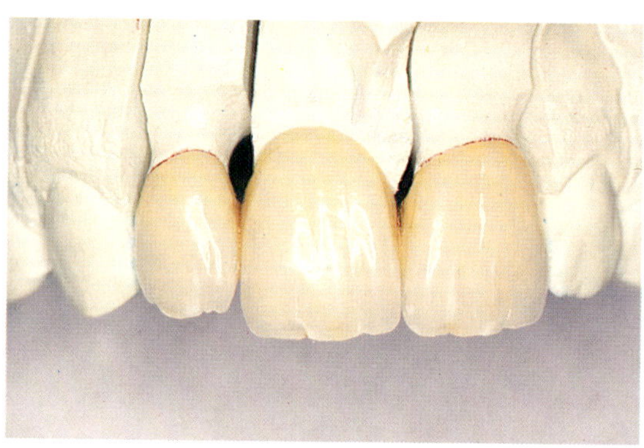

FIG 17–31

The clinical and technological progression from abutment preparation to bridge cementation must be rigidly controlled so that it results clinically in a passive, stable, and simultaneous adaptation of all porcelain margins over the abutments.

Root reproduction lends itself very well to the shoulder porcelain technic when the tooth preparation is adequate. Selection of the adequate cervical tonality allows for optimum translucency without any surface colorant on this maxillary first premolar used as a bridge retainer (Fig 17–32).

GOLD CERAMIC MARGINS

The metal collar provides for porcelain support along the margins. As it is reduced to a hairline, it becomes increasingly difficult to achieve good cervical fit without overcontour since metal, opaque, and porcelain must all terminate over the labial shoulder edge. It is common to prescribe for esthetic reasons a hairline metal collar when a porcelain margin cannot be used, but it still must overcome the gray oxidation line with its shadowing effect and the brightness of the overlying opaque. Application over the cervical area of a mixture of a high gold content paste formulated with a ceramic additive (e.g., Degussa Deckgold, Normal no. 25380010) creates a pleasing esthetic result. This gold bonding agent masks the gray oxidation line and lowers value with a warm golden tone and allows for the reproduction of a root area under minimum thickness.

The first opaque is fired and establishes bonding to the metal coping (Fig 17–33). The gold bonding agent is carefully stirred with one to two drops of the

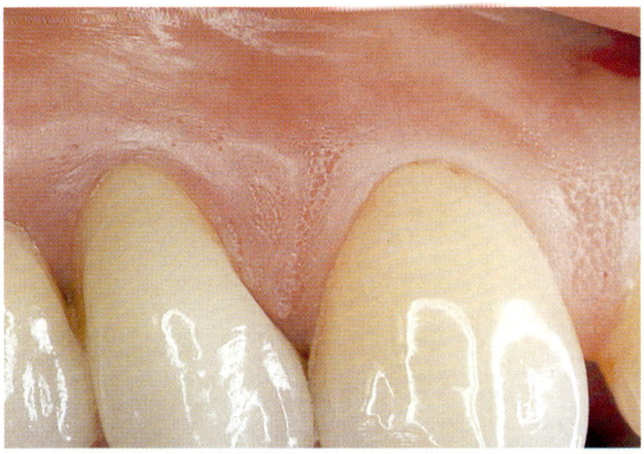

FIG 17–32

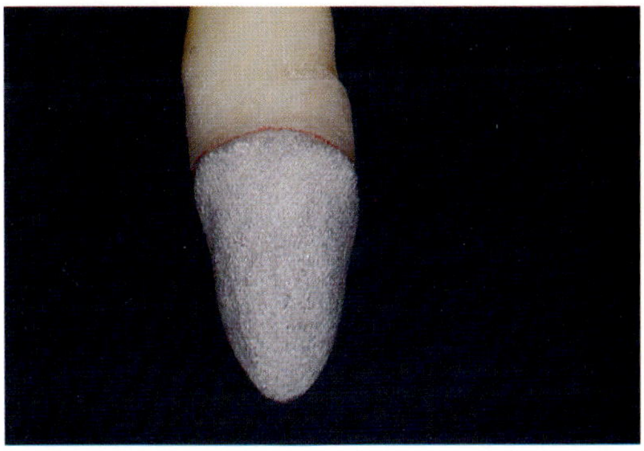

FIG 17–33

supplied liquid to a creamy consistency. It is painted on the cervical area in a very thin coat (Fig 17–34). These agents are claimed by some manufacturers to be 10 to 15 μ thick after firing. It is predried at the muffle entrance for 10 minutes and fired at a rate of 60°C/minute without vacuum from 600°C to 970°C to fuse it to the opaque layer. The bright gold color should be obtained right upon firing (Fig 17–35). If it is darker or dull looking, it means that the firing temperature was too low. The second opaque coat is applied as described in Chapter 2. In essence, the gold ceramic margin acts as a uniquely modified opaque (Fig 17–36).

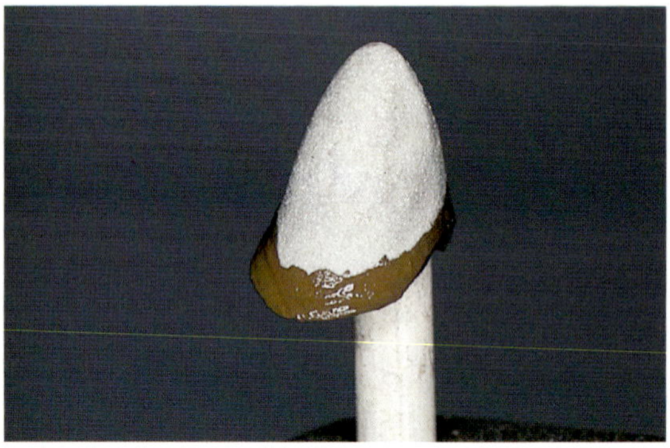

FIG 17–34

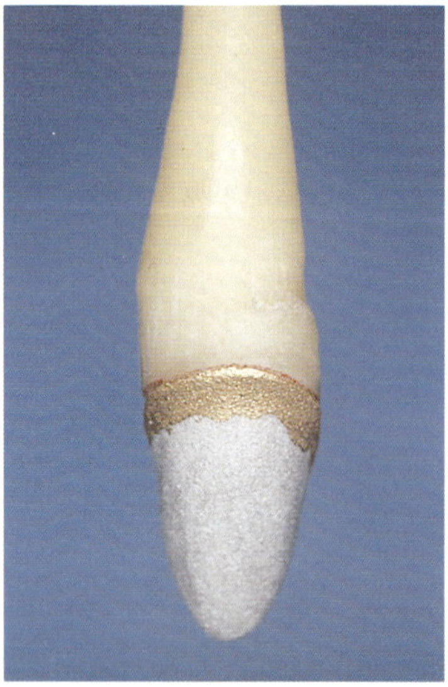

FIG 17–35

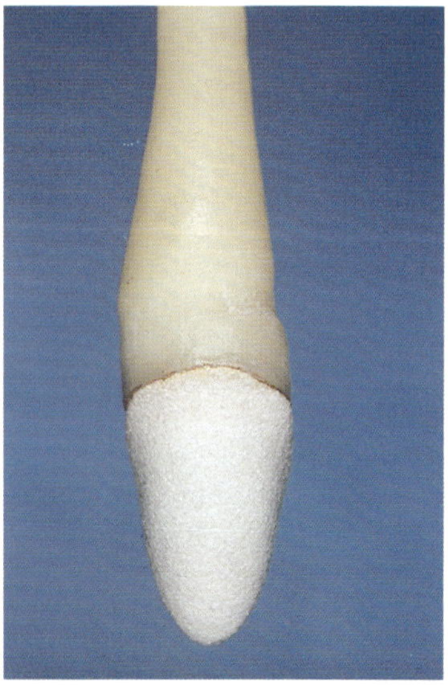

FIG 17–36

Pleasing cervical characteristics are maintained in the finished crown. The metal collar is less conspicuous, and the cervical margin may assume a slightly warmer tone (Fig 17–37).

Root reproduction is accomplished in this situation under a porcelain thickness of 0.8 mm to avoid overcontour. The gold ceramic margins are instrumental in reducing opaque brightness (Figs 17–38 and 17–39).

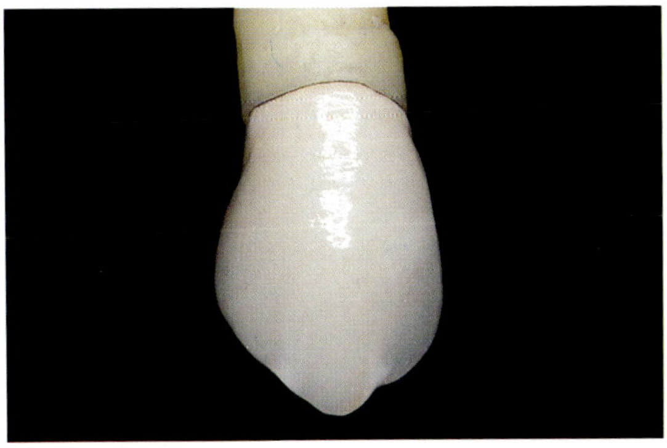

FIG 17–37

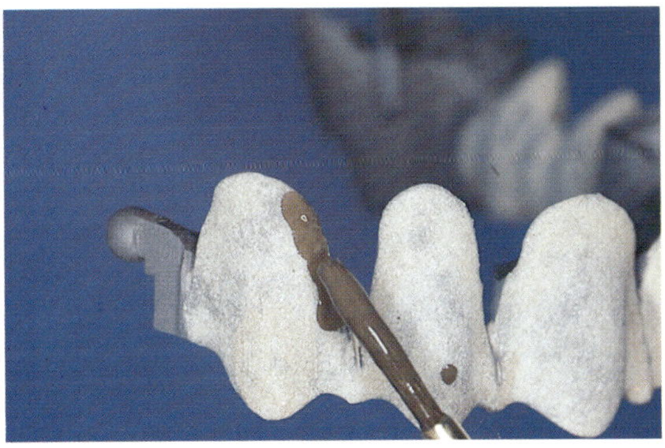

FIG 17–38

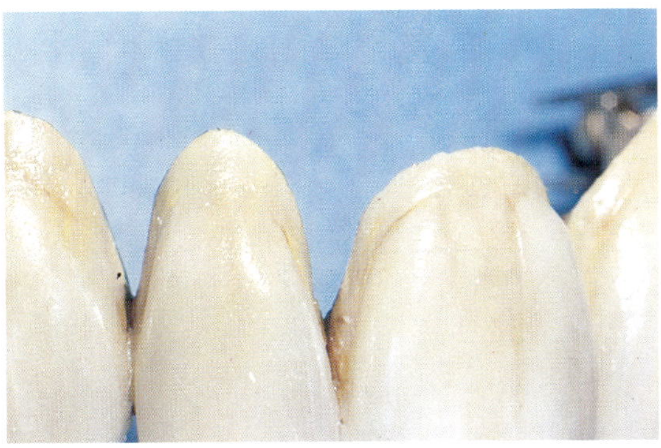

FIG 17–39

REFERENCES

1. Chiche G: Clinical retrospective of porcelain butt margins using high fusing porcelains. Paper presented at the American Academy of Esthetic Dentistry Annual Meeting, Colorado Springs, Colo, 1986.
2. Goldstein RE: Esthetic principles for ceramo-metal restorations. *Dent Clin North Am* 1977; 21:803.
3. Goodacre CH, et al: The collarless metal-ceramic crown. *J Prosthet Dent* 1977; 38:615–622.
4. Schneider DM, Levi MS, Mori DF: Porcelain shoulder adaptation using direct refractory dies. *J Prosthet Dent* 1976; 36:583–587.
5. Sozio RB, Riley DJ: A precision ceramic-metal restoration with a facial butted margin. *J Prosthet Dent* 1977; 37:517–521.
6. Toogood GD, Archibald JF: Technique for establishing porcelain margins. *J Prosthet Dent* 1978; 40:464.
7. Vryonis P: Improving esthetics in porcelain fused to gold restorations *J Prosthet Dent* 1980; 44:667–669.
8 LaHoste LH: The porcelain butt margin. *Quintessence Dent Technol* 1981; 5:149–151.
9. West AJ, Goodacre CJ, Moore BK, et al: A comparison of four techniques for fabricating collarless metal ceramic crowns. *J Prosthet Dent* 1985; 54:5.
10 Cooney JP, Richter WA, MacEntee MI: Evaluation of ceramic margins for metal-ceramic restorations. *J Prosthet Dent* 1985; 54:1.
11. Wanserski DJ, Sobczak KP, Monaco JG, et al: An analysis of margin adaptation of all porcelain facial margin ceramometal crowns. *J Prosthet Dent* 1986; 56:3.
12. Bridger DV, Nicholls JI: Distortion of ceramometal fixed partial dentures during the firing cycle. *J Prosthet Dent* 1981; 45:507.

Index